China's Cancer Solution

What the Chinese Know About Reishi Mushroom That Could Save American Lives

Sharon Brucato

First Edition

7 Day Health
Health Supplements 7 Days a Week

7 Day Health Publishing, Hacienda Heights, California USA

China's Cancer Solution

Sharon Brucato

Editorial Coordinator: Alex Yu

Published by:
7 Day Health
Hacienda Heights, California U.S.A.
reishi@7dayhealth.com

Visit our website: www.alternative2cancer.com

Library of Congress Control Number: 2005906731

Library of Congress Cataloging-in-Publication Data
Brucato, Sharon.
China's cancer solution: what the Chinese know about reishi mushroom that could save American lives / Sharon Brucato; foreword by Daniel Sliva.
p. cm.
Includes bibliographical references and index.
ISBN 0-977-22190-3
1. Health. 2. Naturopathy. 3. Medicine, Popular. 4. Mushrooms-Therapeutic use. I. Title.

Printed in China.

10 9 8 7 6 5 4 3 2 1

The information contained in this book is intended for general reference purposes only. This data is not a substitute for professional medical advice and should not be used to diagnose, treat, cure or prevent any disease. Before starting any new treatment, please seek the advice of a qualified health professional.

This book is dedicated to American cancer victims
Maddi, Cecily and Simon,
who would have suffered less and lived longer
if we'd had this information earlier.

China's Cancer Solution

Contents

China's Cancer Solution

About the Author

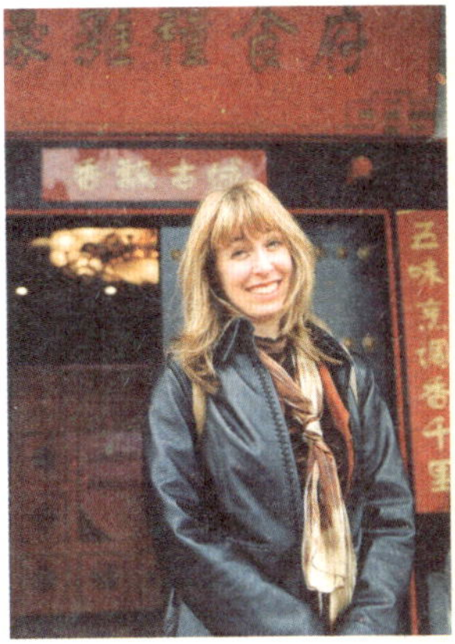

Sharon Brucato has served as a coveted writer for health experts and technologists since 1983. By focusing on new discoveries, she has had the privilege to introduce some of the most useful health and computer products developed in the last 20 years. These include advances in herbal medicine, computer networking and data storage. Brucato has ghostwritten books, feature articles and publicity materials for more than 50 companies in the U.S., Western Europe and now China.

Brucato gained experience as a writer while working for Burson-Marsteller, still one of the world's largest public relations firms. There she was introduced to the excitement of writing and publicity for innovative health and technology corporations. Throughout her career, she has served as a staff and freelance writer for various PR agencies, earning multiple trophies, certificates and commendations for new-product introductions, marketing communications achievement and service to the profession.

As a native of Southern California, Brucato was educated at UCLA, where she earned a bachelor of arts in English. She also attended UCI, where she became certified as a teacher of secondary English and took graduate courses in public relations. Brucato was a law student for two years before marrying her New England-born husband Paul. In 2003, she became one of the first to be certified as a Professional Book Writer (P.B.W.). The author and her husband reside in Southern California with their two children, Alee and Tommy. The family has numerous pets, most notably their beloved Shih Tzu named Reishi!

Foreword

China's Cancer Solution describes the history and use of reishi mushroom for cancer treatment. It is an excellent example of the symbiosis between Traditional Chinese Medicine and Western medicine.

Because cancer is a leading cause of death in the United States, new cancer therapies are of particular importance for cancer patients. Western medicine relies mainly on surgery, radiation therapy and chemotherapy. In addition, pharmaceutical companies are spending billions of dollars for the development of new cancer drugs annually.

However, despite all the money and effort, progress in the development, laboratory testing, and clinical testing of new cancer drugs is sometimes slow, while the population in need of proper cancer treatment is growing. Therefore, alternative therapies have been sought.

Even though a number of natural products have demonstrated scientifically proven anti-cancer effects on cancer cells in laboratory or animal experiments, these natural products are usually ignored or not understood for cancer treatment by Western medicine. On the other hand, a large number of cancer patients focus their hopes for treatment on a variety of dietary supplements. Some of them may work, some of them may not, and some of them may even have negative effects.

Therefore, *China's Cancer Solution* comes just at the right time, when modern scientific methods can demonstrate the anti-cancer effect of reishi on cancer cells at the molecular level, and can scientifically justify the use of an ancient medicinal mushroom for the treatment of cancer patients.

This book will help readers understand the integration of Traditional Chinese Medicine into Western medicine. Most importantly, this book can help patients with their choice of treatment.

Daniel Sliva, Ph.D.
Director, Cancer Research Laboratory
Methodist Research Institute and Department of Medicine
Indiana School of Medicine
Indianapolis, Indiana

Acknowledgments

I am deeply indebted to my newfound friends in China, who generously and expediently shared this lifesaving information with me. I send a special, heartfelt appreciation to the following teams:

Shanghai, China

Mr. Song Tao Lü, founder and chairman of Green Valley Holding Co., Ltd.; a "true man"
Alex Yu, an earnest and down-to-earth man, without whom this book would not have been possible
Dr. Jinshen Chen, inventor of SunRecome, a genius and a very patient man to answer my myriad questions
Daniel Tan, highly capable, tireless professional translator
Hansen Yung, versatile coordinator of head-spinning details
Xue Ren Wang (a.k.a. "Go Fish"), a world-class writer and photographer
Cui Wei Guan, extraordinary female sales director
Professor Zhihong Li, compassionate advocate of integrative medicine who made the data understandable

Huangshan and Xi'an, China

Cailin Liu, vice governor of Huangshan; a generous host
Shi Min Zhou, remarkable director of the SunRecome manufacturing plant

Beijing, China

Dr. Feng Wang, impressive, ultra-professional director of the SunRecome clinical trials
Professor Zhi-Bin Lin, world expert on reishi and a patient man
Professor Mingda Huang, an insightful resource and remarkable inventor of integrative medicine

U.S.A.

Margie Haley, diligent editor and dear friend in Christ

Dr. Daniel Sliva, prolific U.S. reishi expert; immensely and joyfully helpful in clarifying comparative data

Dr. Paul McGlynn, consulting physician

American Cancer Society's Office of Corporate Communications for their rapid assistance

North American Mycological Association (NAMA) for excellent resource information

The Brucato and Howard Families, namely Paul, Alee, Tommy, Leonard and Harriet, who lovingly provided me endless moral support throughout this project

Preface

I have lost too many friends to cancer. You probably have, too. I am tired of hearing about how excruciating and debilitating cancer treatment is in the U.S. You're probably frustrated and unnerved about cancer therapy, also. Does it really make sense to attack cancer cells so ferociously with chemotherapy and radiation that patients have no immune-fighting abilities left to survive the therapy? Surely, there must be a more humane treatment approach!

Approximately 1,500 Americans die of cancer each day, reports the American Cancer Society in its January 19, 2005 release of cancer statistics. Now that Americans have the highest cancer incidence worldwide, it is clear that the U.S. has a problem that it can't adequately address.

While grieving over the grim state of cancer in America, I was contacted by a Chinese company named Green Valley. This ultra-high-tech firm was seeking a U.S. writer to author a book on herbal cancer therapy. I balked. What a waste of time that project would be! Americans are suspicious of China. They don't understand the culture. And they don't believe in herbal therapy. Besides, how can any herb have much effect on cancer? And if there were such a treatment, surely Americans would know about it! My bias, fear and blind disbelief kept me from considering Green Valley's offer.

But my friends and their friends were still dying of cancer — and at an alarming rate. And it seemed as if everyone was living in fear of the "C" word, just as The Gallup Organization reported in its December 2003 headline, *"Americans Worry Most About Getting Cancer."* How could I ignore the possibility that, just maybe, this Chinese company had a better solution to cancer than America did?

I decided that if Green Valley's product could help one family member or friend or acquaintance, then the writing project would, indeed, be worthwhile. So, after surprisingly good preliminary findings about Green Valley's claims, I accepted the offer to write a book about China's cancer solution. As part of the negotiations, Green Valley agreed to allow me access to any expert and any document I required to substantiate their claims. They kept to this agreement, completely and wholeheartedly.

In fact, though I have served as a writer for some of the most innovative health and technology inventors in the U.S., I can state without reservation that none has developed a product as remarkable or life-saving as the concentrated reishi mushroom extract described in this book.

What did I learn from my 47 interviews throughout Southeast China? A profound truth: Green Valley has, indeed, developed an innovative, humane solution to the treatment of cancer. Their herbal product, based on the most revered medicinal mushroom in the world, minimizes radiochemotherapy side effects. And it works alongside chemotherapy and radiation protocols, bringing out the best in Eastern and Western medicine. In short, it cuts cancer down at the cellular level by starving it — without harming healthy cells and while repairing damaged cells. Though this herbal formulation cannot cure every case of cancer, it is, by far, the best adjuvant therapy currently available.

Are you skeptical? I was, too, until I met with leading experts on reishi mushroom, integrative medicine, Traditional Chinese Medicine, pharmacology and molecular biology, plus clinicians and patients. Their data was wholly consistent.

If you or a loved one is suffering from cancer, I hope you will consider the possibility that China has a more humane and effective treatment solution than our own beloved USA does. After all, China's system of medicine is more than 2,500 years old; ours is just over 200 years old. Maybe the Chinese do know something about cancer therapy that we don't!

May God speed healing to every American suffering from cancer.

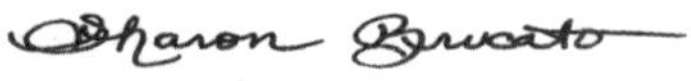

Sharon Brucato

Chapter One

What Americans Don't Know About Cancer Therapy

IN CHINA, CANCER PATIENTS ARE breezing through chemotherapy and radiation treatments, successfully beating back tumor growth, and living in confidence that cancer will not return. Their secret? A high concentration of a medicinal mushroom called reishi, otherwise known as *Ganoderma lucidum* or *ling zhi.*

Reishi is not well known in the United States. If it were, cancer would not have recently displaced heart disease as the leading killer of Americans.[1] And radiochemotherapy would not be debilitating so many patients in the process of treating them. Instead, most American patients would win their war against cancer and, in the process, experience few side effects from Western cancer drugs. This is possible when reishi mushroom and radiochemotherapy are used simultaneously.

What's the Secret Recipe?

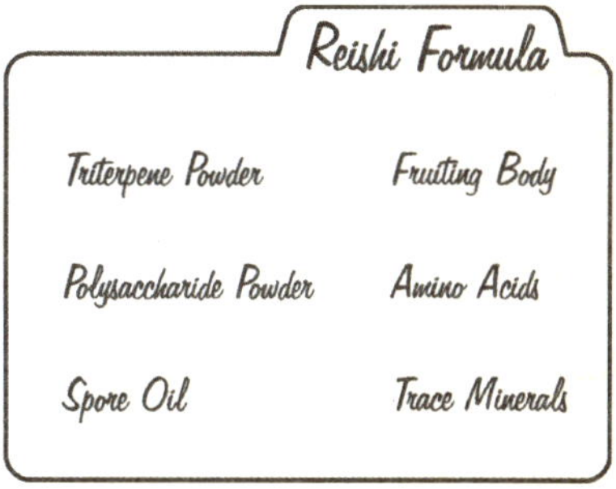

In the U.S., reishi products are available now in the form of coffees, teas, tinctures and capsules. These are nutritional supplements, which are useful preventive measures against the onset of cancer, but they are not powerful enough to combat active cancer, attack its root cause, or suppress radiochemotherapy side effects.

Chinese cancer patients—more than one million of them to date—have used a reishi formulation created through analysis of the mushroom's DNA, from which two key molecules are extracted and concentrated, one 1,000 times, the other 20 times.

Then these molecules, called triterpenes and polysaccharides, are released by pulverizing the reishi mushroom's fruiting body and by subjecting reishi's spores to high-frequency sound waves. When dried, ground, mixed, sterilized and scientifically proportioned, the resulting product is more potent against cancer than any other reishi formulation and any other herbal extract— alone or in combination![2]

Is Reishi a Well-Guarded Secret?

This reishi mushroom formulation is not a new discovery:

- It was created in 1996.
- It became commercially available in 1997.
- It was patented nationwide in China in 2000.[3]
- It was approved in 2002 for use in conjunction with radiochemotherapy by China's FDA (SFDA).[4]
- It was successfully tested from 2001 to 2005 in the world's largest clinical trial of this Traditional Chinese Medicine. *(Please see Chapter 8 for more information.)*
- In March 2005, the United States FDA approved commencement of human studies on SunRecome as an Investigational New Drug. When the clinical trial begins, details will be posted at www.clinicaltrials.gov.

So how is it possible for savvy Americans to be unaware of a cancer treatment that has been successful in China for eight years? There are many reasons, which together explain why this life-saving information comes so late to the U.S.

Why Americans Don't Know

Geographic Distance

In more ways than one, China and America are on opposite sides of the world. Those who brave the distance must travel 6,485 miles one-way. The nonstop journey from Los Angeles takes a grueling 13-½ hours to reach Shanghai, the most populous city. Travel to the next major city, Xi'an, requires an additional two-hour flight for sightseeing in the ancient capital. Two more hours in the air are needed to reach Beijing, today's capital and the location of the 2008 Olympics.

Travel within China is arduous, too, especially for the vast majority of Americans who do not speak or read Chinese and are unfamiliar with the driving habits, pedestrian patterns, bicycle traffic, and cuisine—which is far removed from American Chinese food.

Language Barrier

> 现代医学对癌细胞凋亡的认识为: 癌细胞与衰老是在细胞凋亡 (apoptosis, Apo) 又称细胞程序死亡 (programmed cell death, PCD) 也是在调节机制的控制下。

Those who are familiar with this Chinese text may have previously read it in the 1994 landmark technical paper detailing how concentrated reishi mushroom can affect cancer. But the majority of Americans cannot speak or read Chinese, and most Chinese older than 30 cannot read English. This landmark Chinese paper was not translated into English until 2000.

Eastern Versus Western Medicine

Though Eastern and Western medicines originate from herbs, their end products look vastly different. Doctors of Traditional Chinese Medicine dispense raw or powdered herbs; Western doctors prescribe capsules, tablets, caplets, pills, liquids and patches that derive from herbs—or imitate the function of herbs through synthetic processes.

Philosophically, Eastern and Western medicine are dissimilar, too. Practitioners of Eastern medicine believe that healing is accomplished when the root, the source, the origin of the problem is identified and attended to. This philosophy contrasts sharply with Western medicine, which attacks the symptoms, the outbreak, the physical manifestation of the illness. Simply put, Eastern medicine is holistic, addressing the entire body as one system; Western medicine focuses on body parts.

Yet Chinese medicine is considered quackery by many Western-trained doctors, even though Americans have shown great interest in natural health techniques. In fact, most Americans that undergo treatment for cancer also use some sort of complementary or alternative medicine, according to a 2000 study conducted by the University of Texas-Houston School of Public Health.[5] Still, Western oncologists and radiologists are highly resistant to consult on cases with Eastern-trained practitioners. As a result, cancer patients are reluctant to mention their use of natural medicine to Western-trained doctors.

Regardless, interest in natural medicine is unstoppable. In March 2005, the world's largest natural health trade show—Natural Products Expo West—attracted more than 2,590 exhibitors and 38,000 attendees to its Southern California event.[6] The show's producer reports seeing better science and manufacturing quality every year.

There is more good news: combined Eastern/Western medical teams are beginning to form, thanks to a new healthcare sector called integrative medicine. This practical approach to healthcare integrates Eastern and Western therapies, not as equal halves, but as each therapy is appropriate for the patient. The number of U.S. hospitals offering integrative medical services has more than doubled in the last seven years, because of patient demand.[7]

U.S. hospitals that do offer integrative cancer therapies most often employ acupuncture, chiropractic, homeopathy, dietary modification, exercise regimens, massage, herbal medicine or a combination of these. But China has proven that the most effective integration to date is a particular herbal therapy, namely reishi mushroom, plus radiochemotherapy —a combination that is absent from U.S. integrative hospital care.

No Economic Incentive

The first formula for concentrated reishi mushroom was developed by a scientist working in a government-owned laboratory in China. He had no economic incentive to commercialize the invention, because profits would be retained by the "State," as the Chinese government is called, not by the scientist. And the State had no economic incentive to export the

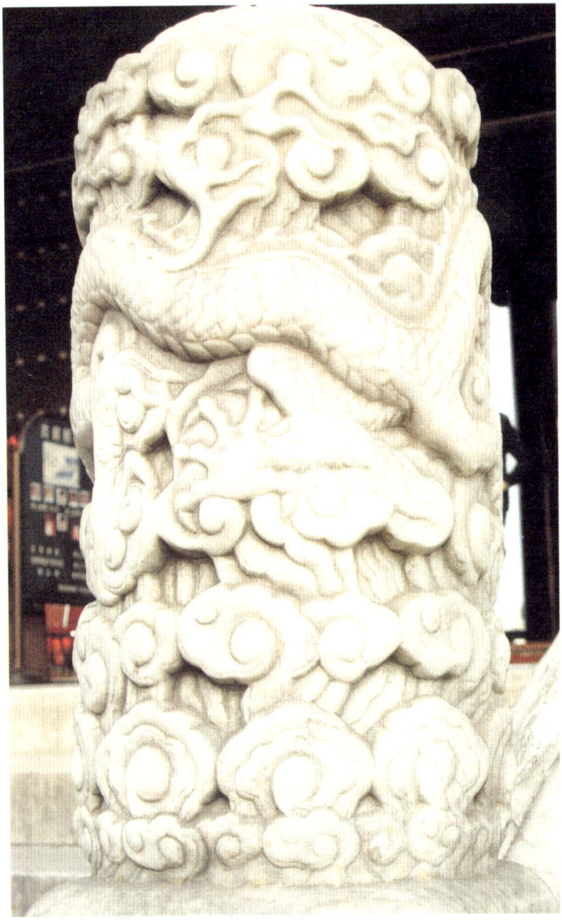

Massive carved reishi column at the Forbidden City

invention to the U.S., which to this day has been slow to accept the 2,500-year-old tradition of Chinese medicine.

It was not until 1996, when capitalism was allowed to flourish in China that a mass market for concentrated reishi was sought within the State, and not until 2004 before U.S. export began.

Cultural Differences

China abounds with art, architecture and advertising depicting the reishi mushroom as a symbol of health and longevity. Americans who travel to China will see these symbols—but they will not likely recognize them. Try this experiment: Ask any Chinese-born American over age 30 what "ling zhi" (pronounced ling-ja') means, and more often than not, the response will be that ling zhi is the herb of immortality, a healing herb, an herb for cancer. Ask any non-Asian U.S. citizen what ling zhi or reishi is (pronounced rē'shē). The response will be, more often than not, a blank stare. Reishi is the most revered herb in the history of Chinese medicine, yet Americans remain unfamiliar with its history and healing potential.

American Bias

Americans readily accept importation of a plethora of goods made in China. In fact, according to the May 9, 2005 issue of *Newsweek*,[8] exports to the United States from China have increased 1,600 percent in the past 15 years. Still, Americans are reluctant to value Chinese medicine, though it is more proven than Western medicine by at least 2,000 years. Americans seem to have a bias against Chinese medicine, blindly adopting the opinions of those held by the Western medical establishment, whose practitioners have rarely taken even one course in the subject.

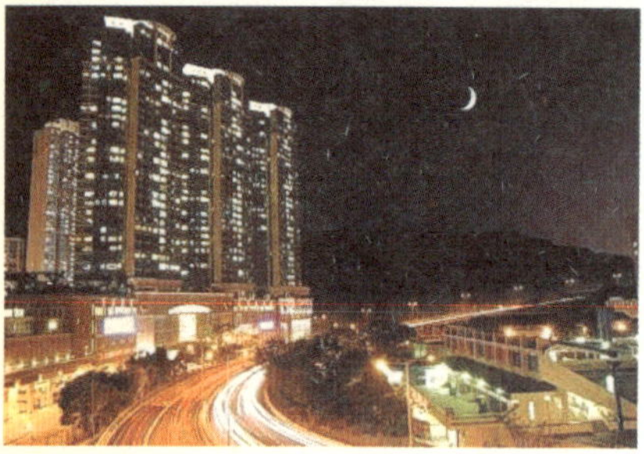

Xi'an's nighttime skyline

China Today

China is a vast country that is undergoing rapid and profound growth and development. Its major cities boast architectural masterpieces of a variety not yet seen in the United States. Travel from the Xi'an or Beijing airports to the business districts feels like a futuristic journey, unparalleled in the variety of skyscrapers, lighting effects, bridges and road design.

Some of the greatest inventions in the world were made by the Chinese. These include:

Chinese Inventions

- Abacus
- Acupuncture
- Book Shops
- Movable Type
- Paper
- Planetarium

Books
Compass
Fan
Fireworks
Gunpowder
Ink
Kites
Printing
Processed Grain
Rudder
Silk
Spaghetti
Traditional Chinese Medicine
and...

...herbal medicine, which may be China's greatest gift of all, especially for those suffering from cancer.

Erase the images of old China, with its gray-suited pedestrians and peasants carrying buckets of rice on sticks across their backs. Think of China as it is today: a technologically advanced society with a deep medical history that Americans have yet to unearth.

In the fight against cancer, Americans must abandon all biases and barriers against China. It is time to take a close look at their most revered herb—reishi mushroom.

Notes

Chapter Two

How Can a Mushroom Affect Cancer?

REISHI IS CATEGORIZED AS A fungus, which is simply the Latin word for mushroom. Worldwide, there are more than 100,000 known species of fungi—some edible, some medicinal and some toxic. But in the U.S., the word "fungus" often carries a negative connotation, evoking images of toadstools, decomposing food, or hippie hallucinogens (those "magic mushrooms" of the '60s and '70s.)

Americans simply do not enjoy fungi as Asians and Europeans do. In China, Japan and France, for example, it is common to see pushcart vendors selling a variety of edible and medicinal wild fungi. But in America, consumers are content to buy their fungi in supermarkets, which mostly sell the ubiquitous *Agaricus bisporus*, better known as the button mushroom and related crimini and portabella.

And relatively few Americans have been known to travel hundreds of miles through forests, fields and mountains in search of rare fungi. But "mushrooming" has been popular throughout Europe and Asia for thousands of years.

Europeans, in particular, delight in hunting for subterranean fungi, known as truffles. This "sport" can yield big payoffs, especially if *Tuber melanosporum* is found. It is worth $800 to $1,500 a pound, making it the world's most expensive mushroom.[9]

Today's Pharmaceuticals Contain Fungi

American pharmaceutical companies know the value of fungi, too, because historically the most common ingredient in Western medicine is—fungus![10] Penicillin, developed in 1928, was obtained from a fungus; today, more than 1,500 antibiotics are produced by fungi (Cephalosporin and tetracycline, for example). Fungus is also a key ingredient in anti-rejection drugs for organ transplants (Cyclosporin); in high-cholesterol medications (Lovastatin); and in steroids for both inflammation (cortisone and prednisone) and oral contraceptives.

How Many Medicinal Fungi Are There?

Mushroom experts, called mycologists, have identified more than 300 medicinal fungi worldwide for use in the prevention or treatment of a wide variety of ailments, including these:

Autoimmune conditions: allergies, asthma, arthritis, dermatitis, diabetes, fibromyalgia, lupus, multiple sclerosis

Weakened immunity: bronchitis, cancer, colds, fever and flu, hepatitis, viruses

Other common ailments: high cholesterol, diarrhea, gastritis, hemorrhoids, high-blood pressure, indigestion, insomnia, muscle spasms, nervousness, poor vision, ulcers, urinary-tract infections

How Can Fungi Aid So Many Conditions?

Fungi are genetically and biochemically different than all other living organisms on earth. For many years, scientists listed fungi in the Plant Kingdom. Then they discovered that fungi have a closer relationship to animals than plants. But they are neither plant nor animal, because fungi:

- do not contain chlorophyll
- are not dependent on light
- cannot produce their own food through photosynthesis
- cannot move from their original location without growing or being transported by wind, water or external forces.

Thus, fungi are classified as their own Kingdom.[11]

The Kingdom Fungi is one of God's most fascinating creations. Fungi can grow on all continents, in all climates, in every season of the year, in every color, in more shapes than can be classified, and in sizes ranging from microscopically visible to as much as 150 pounds. They can be found in soil, on living and dead plants, on rocks, insects, animals, people, or floating in the air or water. Fungi seem to appear from nowhere after the rain and in dark, damp places. They have no leaves, no seeds and no discernable roots.

Though many people think that fungi offer no nutritional value, the opposite is true. Fungi are packed with biochemical properties, including:

- Protein
- Fiber
- Amino acids
- Vitamins A, B-complex, C and D
- Minerals including copper, iron, niacin, phosphorus, potassium, riboflavin and selenium.[12]

These nutrients help the human body maintain normal heart rhythm, fluid balance, muscle and nerve function, contribute to the health of the immune, thyroid and male reproductive systems, provide antioxidants to fight cell-damaging free radicals, help produce red blood cells, and release energy from the fat, protein and carbohydrates in food.

Fungi For Cancer Treatment

Scientists have also discovered more than 300 species of fungi that can activate the immune system and inhibit the growth of tumors. Consistent use of medicinal fungi has been associated with a lower death rate from cancer, according to a 14-year-long survey conducted among Japanese mushroom workers in the Nagano Prefecture. There, the average cancer death rate dropped from one in 600 farmers to one in 1,000 farmers who consumed medicinal fungi.[13]

Fungi offering the greatest promise for cancer therapy are:

Agaricus (Himmematsutake)	*Agaricus blazei*
Chaga	*Inonotus obliquus*
Cordyceps	*Cordyceps sinensis*
Maitake (Hen of the Woods)	*Grifola frondosa*
Oyster	*Pleurotus ostreatus*

Reishi	*Ganoderma lucidum*
Shiitake	*Lentinulu edodes*

These cancer-fighting fungi have attracted scientific attention because they each contain a high concentration of polysaccharides, a medicinal compound that stimulates the immune system. Polysaccharides are complex sugars made up of thousands of individual molecules. One of the most important polysaccharide is called beta glucan. It stimulates human cells to mobilize an army of messengers called cytokines, which boost the immune system in the following ways:

- T cells —improve immune surveillance
- Natural-Killer Cells (NK cells) — identify and deactivate dysfunctional body cells
- Tumor-Necrosis Factors (TNF) — reduce cell adhesions
- Interferon —immune stimulator
- Interleukins —stimulate antibody production

According to SupplementWatch, Inc., the NK cells stimulated by reishi polysaccharides are especially valuable in cancer therapy. This watchdog group of scientists, physiologists, nutritionists and other health professionals exists to educate people about the pros and cons of dietary supplementation. They say:

> "Reishi has been shown to be a useful adjuvant treatment against cancer when combined with radiation and chemotherapy. This cancer-specific effect of reishi, in addition to its general properties as a broad-spectrum immune modulator (like echinacea) may be due to the findings that reishi polysaccharides can increase numbers and activity of a particular class of immune system cells known as Natural Killer cells (NK cells). These NK cells are particularly active in identifying and deactivating dysfunctional body cells, such as those undergoing unchecked growth."[14]

Of all the fungi, reishi has the highest concentration of polysaccharides—up to 40 percent more by weight than agaricus, chaga, cordyceps, maitake, oyster or shiitake mushrooms![15] Thus reishi is the best choice for increasing the immune-activating response to cancer cells.

In addition to polysaccharides, reishi contains another vital medicinal compound called triterpenes (ganoderic acids –R, -T, -U, -V, -W, -X, -Y and –Z), which can inhibit the intracellular message for cancer cells to reproduce themselves. Scientific proof was presented as early as 1983, when a team of biochemists revealed that reishi's triterpenes showed anti-tumor activity against liver cancer.[16]

Through its polysaccharides and triterpenes, reishi delivers a one-two punch to cancer by improving overall human immunity while inhibiting tumor growth. Best of all, reishi performs these life-saving functions without toxic side effects, giving it a definitive advantage over any other medicinal therapy for cancer patients.

At first glance, Americans might categorize the above information about mushroom science as "fringe science" and the resulting products as "charlatanism." But the fact remains that the health benefits and medicinal value of mushrooms are well known in other countries and can be verified through thousands of research papers. And of all the mushrooms, reishi is the one that is most valued in Chinese medicine. It is worth a closer look.

Notes

Chapter Three

What's So Special About Reishi?

Reishi Is The Most Revered herb in the history of Chinese medicine. Emperors of every dynasty used it to prolong life, while commoners were forbidden to touch it because of its scarcity. Why was it considered to be so valuable?

- It was reported to heal more ailments than any other herb.
- It was rumored to be completely nontoxic, no matter how long it was used or what food or medicine was consumed with it.

Modern scientific research has proven these long-standing claims to be true! That is why reishi continues to be ranked as the #1 herb in the highest category of Chinese medicine since the third century B.C.[17]

Reishi Myths, Legends & Folklore

As the most powerful and famous Chinese herb, reishi has been immortalized in myths, legends and folklore. The most famous story has been turned into a Beijing Opera, which is the highest standard of opera performed throughout China today. The opera is called "The Legend of the White Snake."[18] This story is so well-known and beloved in China that most adults over 30 years old can retell it.

Here is an Anglicized, abbreviated version:

"Once upon a time there were two magical snakes that turned themselves into beautiful young ladies named Lady White and Lady Green.

One day, they decided to visit West Lake in Hang Zhou because of its famed beauty. There they met a man named Xian Xu. Both Lady White and Xian Xu fell in love at first sight. They married soon afterward and Lady White was with child.

"Soon it became time for the annual Dragon Boat Festival, when Chinese families drank wine to drive away spirits. Lady White knew this was a dangerous time for her, because her pregnancy had weakened her magical powers. When her husband insisted that she drink the wine, she took a sip to please him. Immediately she turned back into a snake, which frightened her husband so that he died.

"When the power of the festival wine wore off, Lady White resumed her human form. She was heartbroken to find her husband dead. *But she knew that the celestial, glossy Ganoderma (lucidum) found on the mountain could bring him back to life.*

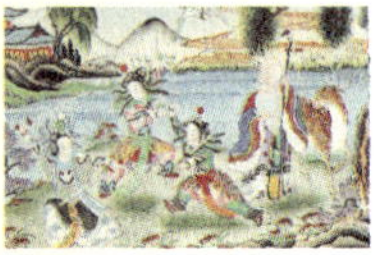

Battle scene from the "White Snake" opera

"Using her magical powers, she flew to the mountain and attempted to steal the herb, but it was surrounded by a white crane and heavenly guards. Lady White fought with the guards and was about to lose the battle when the voice of The Immortal of the South Pole cried out for the fighting to stop. In tears, Lady White begged him to give her the herb. Impressed by her sincerity and true love for her husband, The Immortal granted her request.

"Lady White returned home and ground the herb into a powder. When she gave it to her husband, he returned to life. Lady White and Xian Xu then lived happily ever after with their child."

Reishi's Healing Powers

Though reishi cannot return the dead to life, its reputation as a powerful healing herb is, clearly, quite extensive. Even today, it is referred to as the:

"Elixir of Immortality"

"Herb of Spiritual Potency"

"King of Herbs"

Interestingly, reishi has long been recommended by Chinese herbalists for all kinds of ailments, including:

Altitude sickness	Heart palpitations
Appetite loss	Hepatitis
Arthritis	High cholesterol
Asthma	Hypertension
Chronic bronchitis	Insomnia
Coronary heart disease	Lack of energy
Dermatitis	Migraines
Digestive disorders	Muscle diseases
Dizziness	Nervousness
Eye inflammation	Shortness of breath
Fatigue	Stiff necks/shoulders
Forgetfulness	Tumors

Scientists now know why reishi is reported to aid so many health conditions. This single fungus is endowed with more than 50 polysaccharide molecules and more than 150 triterpene molecules, which together bring the body into balance by increasing immunity better than any other medicinal substance while decreasing cancer cells, viruses, bacteria and protozoa.

Expert Opinions

Leading herbalists agree that reishi has the potential to boost the immune system and fight cancer:

"Animal studies have shown that reishi improves immune function and inhibits the growth of some malignant tumors. It is also a natural anti-inflammatory agent."— **Andrew Weil, M.D., (www.drweil.com), America's best-known naturopath**

"*Ganoderma lucidum* clearly possesses immuno-modulatory and anti-tumor properties."— **Professor Zhi-Bin Lin, "China's Father of Reishi Research," who published the first systematic paper on the subject in 1974**

"*Ganoderma lucidum* has demonstrated strong activity against breast and prostate cancer cells."—**Daniel Sliva, Ph.D., America's foremost expert on reishi and cancer; director of the Cancer Research Laboratory at Methodist Research Institute, Indianapolis, Indiana**

"Today the king of fungi (reishi) is used especially for aging-related and degenerative conditions, such as cancer, and as an immune stimulant."
— Christopher Hobbs, noted American herbalist and botanist (www.christopherhobbs.com), who has studied fungi as medicine for more than 30 years

World Literature

Because of its promising role in cancer treatment, reishi has been the subject of thousands of technical articles published in scientific journals worldwide. One key resource, (www.pubmed.com), contains the most data. Pubmed.com is a service of the U.S. National Institutes of Health (NIH), which maintains the largest medical library in the world. Its collection includes these article titles:

"*Ganoderma lucidum* extracts inhibit growth and induce actin polymerization in **bladder cancer** cells in vitro"— **Cancer Lett. 2004 Dec 8;216(1):9-20.**

"*Ganoderma lucidum* suppresses growth of **breast cancer** cells through the inhibition of Akt/NF-kappaB signaling"— **Nutr Cancer. 2004;49(2):209-16.**

"Effects of *Ganoderma lucidum* on apoptotic and anti-inflammatory function in HT-29 human **colonic carcinoma** cells" — **Phytother Res. 2004 Sep;18(9):768-70.**

"Antitumor and antimetastatic effects on **liver** of triterpenoid fractions of *Ganoderma lucidum*: mechanism of action and isolation of an active substance"— **Anticancer Res. 2002 Nov-Dec;22(6A):3309-18.**

"*Ganoderma lucidum* inhibits proliferation and induces apoptosis in human **prostate cancer** cells PC-3"— **Int J Oncol. 2004 May;24(5):1093-9.**

It is a fact that reishi contains valuable anti-cancer compounds. But scientists caution that the quality of these compounds varies significantly if reishi's exacting growing conditions are not met. The next chapter provides the details.

Notes

Notes

Chapter Four

Where On Earth Does Reishi Come From?

Fungi Are Among The Most difficult agricultural products to cultivate, and reishi ranks as one of the most difficult of all fungi to grow. For medicinal purposes, reishi's growth requirements are even more exacting. Without optimal soil conditions, temperature, air quality, light, moisture, humidity and altitude, its healing properties are rendered weak or impotent.

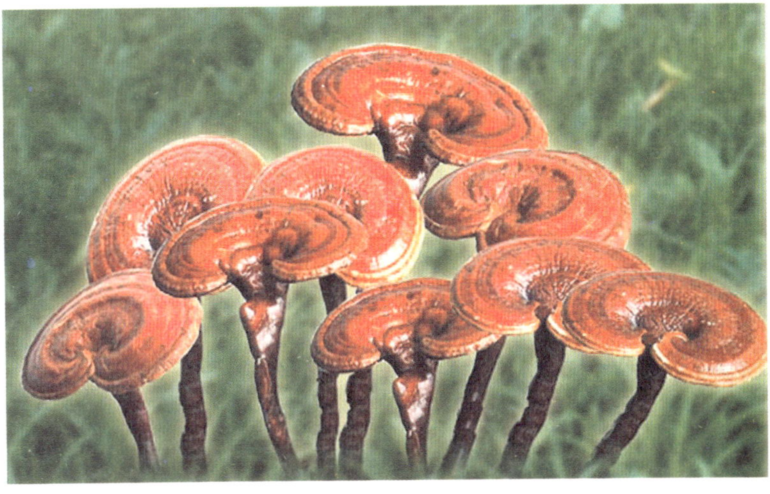

Fully ripe red reishi mushrooms

The reishi fungus itself has a simple, three-part structure: spores, cap, and stem. Its spores can boost the immune system. Its cap and stem, known as the fruiting body, contain polysaccharides and triterpenes that can inhibit the intracellular message that tells cancer cells to reproduce. Growing conditions at all stages of development affect the medicinal value of these three parts.

Spores

The reishi mushroom sprouts from a spore, which contains its reproductive capabilities, much like seeds do, though spores are microscopic. A single reishi mushroom can produce thousands of spores, but they rarely reproduce, because spores have tough, outer husks, which make germination with another spore unlikely. In fact, wild reishi can be found on only two or three of every 10,000 decaying trees, primarily in the mountainous, coastal regions of China.

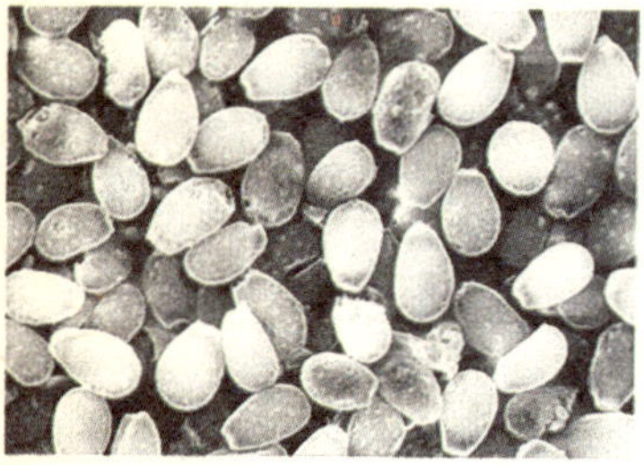
Microscopic view of reishi spores

Cap

If a spore does germinate, it creates an underground network of threads, called mycelia. These mycelia will develop into a mushroom shape, consisting of a stem and cap—if soil conditions offer a pH value of 4.0~6.0. Values higher or lower will limit the size that the cap can grow and the quality of its spore contents.

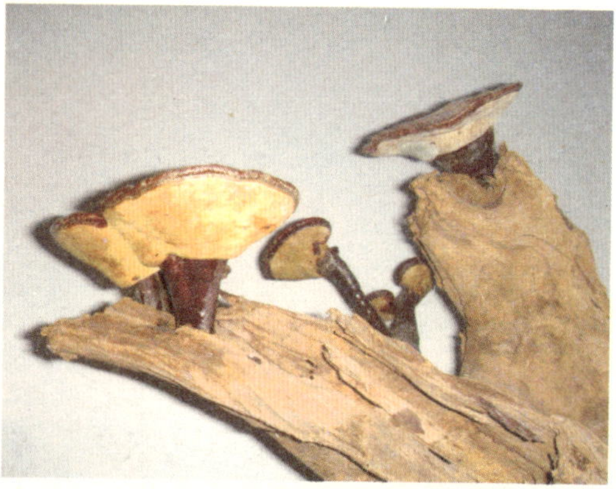
Underside of reishi cap

Other factors affect cap development, including temperature, air quality and light.

Temperature

Reishi flourishes in the range of 75° to 86° F. Higher or lower temperatures stunt or deform cap growth, often into a deer-antler shape, which is ornamental but medicinally useless.

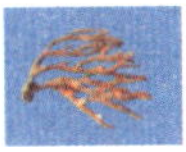

Antler-shaped reishi have no medicinal value.

Air

If carbon dioxide density exceeds 0.1 percent during reishi's growth, its cap will mutate into a deer-antler shape without a cap or spores.

Light

Though some fungi can grow well in total darkness, reishi needs dim light at various stages of its growing cycle to produce the highest quality triterpenes. Too much light will inhibit reishi's growth.

Stem

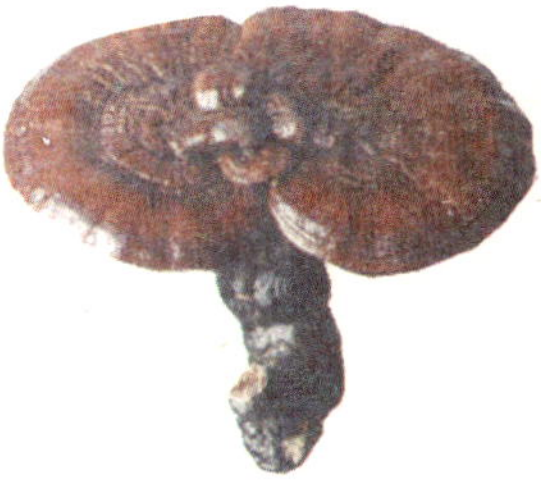

Also known as its stipe, reishi's stem is as hard as wood and has a shiny-red, lacquered ("lucidum") appearance. Stem length and thickness are affected by moisture, humidity and elevation.

Moisture

Reishi requires 60-percent water for hardy stem growth. Too much or too little water will deform the stem or reduce its potential length and width.

Humidity

High humidity is needed through all stages of reishi development. If humidity falls below 80 percent, the reishi fungus will die.

Altitude

Reishi grows best in the forest at high altitudes, no less than half a mile above sea level. That is why it is usually found in mountain ranges.

Reishi's fruiting body has a short life, but its mycelium lives underground for many years, extracting nutrients from its growing medium (soil, wood, etc.) and sending up another fruiting body in two or three years if growing conditions are ideal—which is rare in reishi's natural environment.

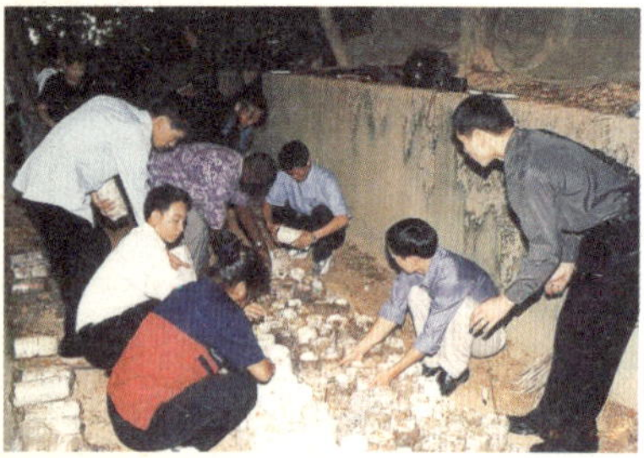

Reishi grown in bottles

Artificial Cultivation

Clearly, wild growth is insufficient to meet the demand for reishi as a multi-use medicine. So in the 1950s and 1960s, Chinese scientists perfected artificial cultivation of reishi. Each fall, they would place reishi spores in ordinary, upright glass bottles layered with sawdust. When the spores germinated, they would transplant the outgrowth

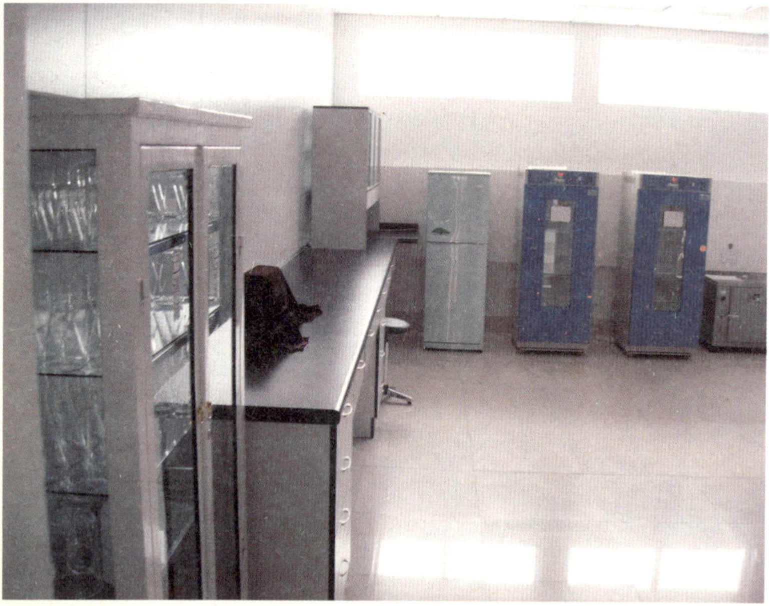

A modern reishi laboratory

(spawn) to hardwood logs from live trees they would chop down. Then they would bury the logs in mud just a few inches below ground and harvest ripe reishi mushrooms in the spring and fall.

But even this method soon fell behind the demand for reishi when, in the 1990s, it became well-known in China that reishi's polysaccharides and triterpenes were powerful cancer fighters.

So mycologists (mushroom scientists) began using other growing mediums, known as substrates. These materials not only enabled mass production of reishi but reduced the need to cut down aged trees. Today reishi is cultivated in:

- Felled and decaying trees
- Wood pulp
- Rice, corn or soybean stalks
- Wheat straw
- Corncobs
- Cottonseed or lotus-seed shells
- Wild grass placed in polyvinyl bags [19]

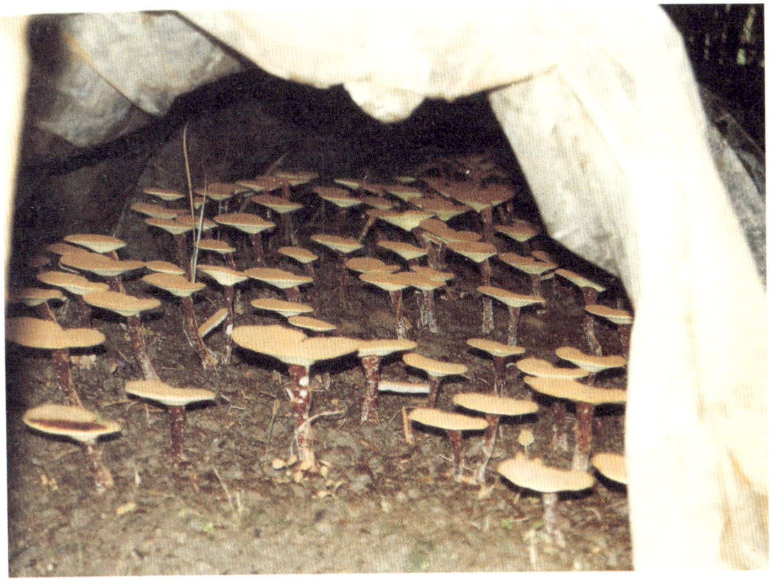

Typical reishi greenhouse

Using a variety of substrates, today's manufacturers can mimic the growing conditions of wild reishi via climate-controlled, sterilized laboratories and specialized greenhouses. These modern practices assuredly supply enough medicinally potent reishi to meet the growing demand.

But just how potent must reishi be to attack cancer cells while protecting healthy cells? The next chapter contains the formula.

Notes

Notes

Chapter Five

How Reishi Starves Cancer Cells

SINCE THE THIRD CENTURY B.C., reishi mushroom has primarily been consumed as a tea, made by drying, grinding and boiling its fruiting body. This simple formula is strong enough to prevent or treat immune-system invasions from bacteria, viruses, protozoa, autoimmune attacks, low-immunity conditions, and a host of other ailments. However, crude reishi powder is not potent enough to deter the progression of cancer.

Still, as early as the 1950s, Asian scientists theorized that reishi held the greatest promise for cancer therapy. But it was not until the 1970s that scientific methods existed to test their theories about reishi's healing mechanisms. That is when the first of four breakthrough experiments occurred, leading to the ability to starve cancer cells with reishi mushroom.

Polysaccharides Indirectly Attack Tumors

The first landmark experiment was conducted by a team of Japanese molecular biologists.[20] They injected reishi polysaccharides into tumorous mice and proved that:

1. Reishi polysaccharides do, in fact, contain anti-tumor properties.
2. Reishi polysaccharides do not directly kill tumors; instead, they stimulate the immune system, which in turn increases its ability to fight off invading cancer cells.

Armed with scientific proof that reishi contained anti-tumor properties, a team of Chinese pharmacologists then conducted the second landmark experiment in the 1970s. They proved that reishi polysaccharides stimulate the *entire* immune system.

Polysaccharides Boost the Entire Immune System

The experiment[21] was developed by "China's Father of Reishi Research," Professor Zhi-Bin Lin. His team lowered the immune system of young and old laboratory mice by forcing them to swim in 57° F water for five minutes. The mice were subjected to this stress test daily for 10 days. A second set of mice was not stressed in any way. Immune system function tests revealed, not surprisingly, that only the first set of mice had impaired immune systems. However, when the scientists injected reishi polysaccharides into the stressed mice, they discovered that after 10 days the immune system functioned normally. This revealed that reishi prevented stress from lowering the immune function.

The results of the 1970 experiments convinced Asian scientists that reishi polysaccharides did, in fact, contain the potential to activate the whole immune system against cancer in humans. Still, scientists had not yet been able to determine the necessary concentration of polysaccharides needed to elevate human immune function to the point that cancer cells could

Zhi-Bin Lin, M.D., O.M.D.
"China's Father of Reishi Research"

- The first to systematically describe reishi's healing properties (1974)
- Recognized internationally for having performed more scientific experiments and published more technical papers about reishi than anyone else in the world
- Former Vice President of Beijing Medical University
- Professor of Pharmacology at Beijing University Since 1971
- President of the Chinese Pharmacological Society (2004)
- First Chinese Board Member of the International Union of Pharmacology
- National Committee Member of the Chinese Association for Science and Technology
- Vice President of the Chinese Edible Fungi Association
- Chairman of the 15th World Pharmacology Conference (2006) in Beijing

no longer survive. And it would be another decade before laboratory equipment could produce high concentrations of reishi's raw materials.

That is when, in 1984, the third experiment took place, this time by a learned Chinese doctor of both Western and Eastern medicine named Jinshen Chen. He derived the potency formula.

Polysaccharides Must be Concentrated 20:1

Using tumorous mice, Dr. Chen injected five times the amount of polysaccharides that naturally occur in reishi mushrooms.[22] The tumors were minimally affected. He increased the dose to 10:1 and 15:1 concentrations. No significant improvement. But when he injected a 20:1 concentration, tumor growth was stunted in the majority of the mice. Dr. Chen further increased the dose to a 30:1 concentration but discovered that it had no greater effect than 20:1—the optimal dose.

Dr. Chen's findings spurred a fourth team of scientists to focus on reishi's other key medicinal compound, triterpenes. What would happen if these were concentrated?

Triterpenes Shrink Tumors and Minimize Chemo Side Effects

In this pivotal 1984 experiment, Chinese scientists[23] injected ever-increasing concentrations of triterpenes into tumorous mice that were being treated with a common chemotherapy drug known as DDP. This drug was known to shrink tumors, but in the process it caused kidney damage, heart palpitations and other side effects. From this study, scientists made two critical observations:

1. Even very small amounts of reishi triterpenes—as little as 15 milligrams—killed tumor cells.
2. Reishi triterpenes minimized the toxic side effects of the chemotherapy drug.

The DDP experiment prompted Dr. Jinshen Chen to put all the pieces of the puzzle together. He contemplated what would happen if reishi's two key medicinal compounds—polysaccharides and triterpenes—were concentrated and injected into tumor cells. Could the cells survive?

For 10 years, Dr. Chen performed in vitro (cellular) and in vivo (animal) studies before discovering how reishi's two key compounds worked in concert to starve tumor cells. In 1994, he published his findings and received commendations from the Traditional Chinese Medicine Association. But China had not been open to the world for very long then, so Dr. Chen's breakthrough paper was not translated into other languages for many years and not into English until 2000.[24]

Here is an excerpt from Dr. Chen's paper, which was the first in the world to explain how to starve cancer cells using concentrated polysaccharides and triterpenes from the reishi mushroom.

Excerpted from the "Pharmacological Function of Reishi for Cancer Prevention," 1994, Hong Kong

"Reishi is universally acknowledged to be one of the most efficacious medicines for cancer prevention and treatment. Why does it have such an effect? Let's analyze the growing laws of cancer cells and normal cells first. Normal cells have a defined lifespan. When new cells are propagated, old cells die naturally. In this way, cells metabolize in a cycle to maintain normal body functions.

"But cancer cells have limitless fertility; a strong and never-ending lifespan. They can destroy normal organic cells by making them lose their function. Research shows this is because of a kind of eternal enzyme inside cancer cells, known as the DNA enzyme.

"Both normal cells and cancer cells have DNA at the end of their chromosomes, which endow filial generation cells and parental generation cells with the same hereditary characteristics. Usually, when cells split, the DNA of normal cells shortens. After dozens of splittings, DNA will deplete and cells will die.

"But cancer cells have the DNA enzyme inside them to protect their DNA from damage when the cells split again and again. This gives cancer cells an endless splitting ability.

"A high-density reishi powder rapidly restricts the growth of cancer cells and reduces the activation of the DNA enzyme. Under microscopic examination of cancer cell tissues, cancer cells will clearly contract and deform, and their tissues will shrink accordingly.

"Reishi destroys cancer DNA enzyme proliferation through its polysaccharides, triterpenes, and other reishi compounds, which penetrate into cancer cells and integrate with the DNA enzyme, thus lengthening the molecule of the enzymes, which changes and destroys their activation.

Once cancer DNA cells lose their protection, they shorten each time they split and gradually die out because they have no splitting abilities."

In essence, Dr. Chen's paper reveals that there is an enzyme in DNA that causes cancer cells, but concentrated reishi triterpenes, polysaccharides and other active compounds suppress these enzymes, which, in turn, starve tumor growth.

Late in 1994, Dr. Chen developed his first reishi anti-tumor formula as a government laboratory scientist. To refine his product and to distribute it widely, it was necessary for Dr. Chen to establish his own pharmaceutical company. He did so and went on to invent a suite of reishi products for chronic bronchitis, diabetes, hypertension, and prostate cancer.

In 1995, the success of Dr. Chen's company attracted the attention of Mr. Song Tao Lü, president of Shanghai Green Valley Holding Company, who had devoted his life to the development of Traditional Chinese Medicine products. His primary interest lay in the reishi mushroom's potential for cancer therapy.

Mr. Lü gave Dr. Chen a very attractive offer: head Green Valley's research and development and establish a world-class reishi laboratory to further refine the high-potency reishi formula. Dr. Chen agreed. Green Valley then created a reishi manufacturing plant in Xian, China, where Dr. Chen turned his original formulation into the most potent reishi extract ever invented.

More than one million cancer patients in China have used Dr. Chen's reishi formulation, which outsells any other reishi product in China, where there are more reishi products than anywhere else in the world. Why is Dr. Chen's formula so successful? Chapter 6 reveals the facts.

Notes

Chapter Six

"Double Excellence"

China Is The World's Primary source of reishi mushrooms and reishi products. More reishi grows wild in China, is cultivated in China, transplanted from China, and sold in China than anywhere else in the world. Yet among at least 100 different formulations, only one reishi product is approved by China's FDA (SFDA) for use in conjunction with chemotherapy and radiation treatments. Since it was introduced in 1997, this formulation has outsold all other reishi products combined, providing assistance to more than one million cancer patients.

What is this notable reishi formulation called? SunRecome™ (pronounced sun'rē-käm). Its name means "double excellence," because the product starves cancer cells and, at the same time, it protects healthy cells and repairs cells damaged by radiochemotherapy and surgery procedures.

SunRecome has met the USFDA's burden of proof as a promising adjuvant cancer therapy. In March 2005, the FDA granted the go-ahead for U.S. clinical trials of SunRecome. This process is expected to commence late in 2005 and can take 10 years to complete. But in the interim, SunRecome is available as a dietary supplement through U.S. distributors.

The Formula

At first glance, SunRecome's formula sounds simple: reishi extract and spore powder. But which of reishi's 50 polysaccharides and which of its 150 triterpene molecules have been extracted to boost human immunity and starve tumor growth? And what is the best concentration of each component?

That is the real secret behind SunRecome's formula, which was invented by Dr. Jinshen Chen. He became the first to:

1) isolate the exact spectrum of reishi triterpenes that can starve tumor cells,

2) determine that a 20:1 potency of reishi polysaccharides is necessary to affect human immunity, and

3) discover that triterpenes work synergistically with other reishi compounds to starve cancer cells and cause their death.

In a 1994 technical article, Dr. Chen explains this interrelationship:

"Cancer cells break down DNA through high levels of two enzymes: topoisomerase and telomerase. Reishi's fruiting body contains naturally occurring molecules, called triterpenes, that slow these cancer enzymes. Because cancer cells have a shorter life span than healthy cells, cancer cells die out (apoptosis) when they are not fed an overabundance of topoisomerase and telomerase. Without negatively affecting healthy cells, reishi triterpenes starve cancer cells.

"In addition to triterpenes in its fruiting body, reishi also contains polysaccharides. These "many sugars" are primarily found inside the spores released under the cap of the mushroom. Reishi polysaccharides increase the white blood cell count (WBC), which boosts the immune system's ability to fight disease.

"It takes a high concentration of polysaccharides and triterpenes, along with reishi's other raw materials, to attack cancer cells, minimize radiochemotherapy side effects and boost the immune system to overcome cancer. But this can be accomplished when:

1. *Reishi's fruiting body is concentrated into a 20:1 reishi powder.*
2. *Spores are collected from the fruiting body at a ratio of 1,000:1.*
3. *The powders consist of reishi triterpenes, polysaccharides, spores, plus 18 amino acids and trace minerals."*

The resulting formula is proprietary; it is SunRecome, the fruit of Dr. Chen's life work exploring—and realizing—the potential of reishi mushroom for cancer therapy.

The Manufacturer

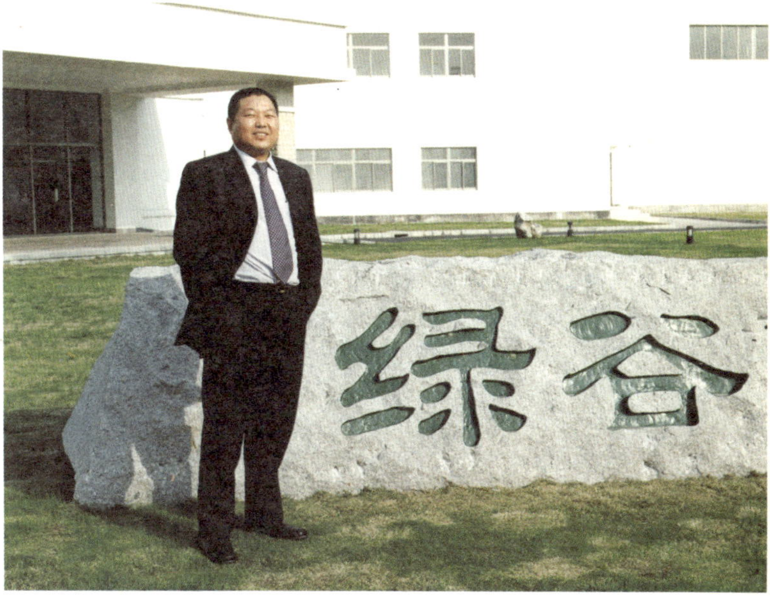

Mr. Song Tao Lü is president of the Green Valley Holding Company, Ltd., manufacturer of SunRecome.

SunRecome is manufactured by the Green Valley Holding Company, Ltd., (www.green-valley.com) based in Shanghai, China. Since it was founded in 1997, Green Valley has earned many honors[25] for its SunRecome product and corporate management under the able leadership of Mr. Song Tao Lü, president and chairman:

- Between 2000 and 2005, Green Valley was named three times as a top 100 private high-technology enterprise.
- The company is listed as a top 50 industrial enterprise, in terms of sales revenue, by the Shanghai Industry Business Bureau, representing the most densely populated manufacturing area of China.

- SunRecome outsells all other reishi products in China.
- Green Valley has earned both ISO 9002 and GMP certification for its quality manufacturing processes.
- SunRecome is the only patented reishi formulation in China!
- This product is the only reishi formulation approved for use by China's FDA as an adjuvant radiochemotherapy treatment.
- SunRecome has been tested in the world's largest clinical trial of reishi mushroom, a Traditional Chinese Medicine.
- In March 2005, the United States FDA granted approval for SunRecome clinical trials to commence as an Investigational New Drug (IND) for oncology.

Green Valley staff credentials are equally as impressive as its product commendations. Eighty-two percent of the company's 4,000 employees hold university degrees. Six hundred employees are medical or pharmaceutical experts. Five hundred are technical personnel.

Green Valley is truly a large company. It maintains 126 branch offices located throughout 29 provinces in China. It manufactures more than 40 different Traditional Chinese Medicine products made in the company's five production facilities. And it is currently creating a worldwide product distribution network, with the goal of promoting modernization of Traditional Chinese Medicine throughout the world.

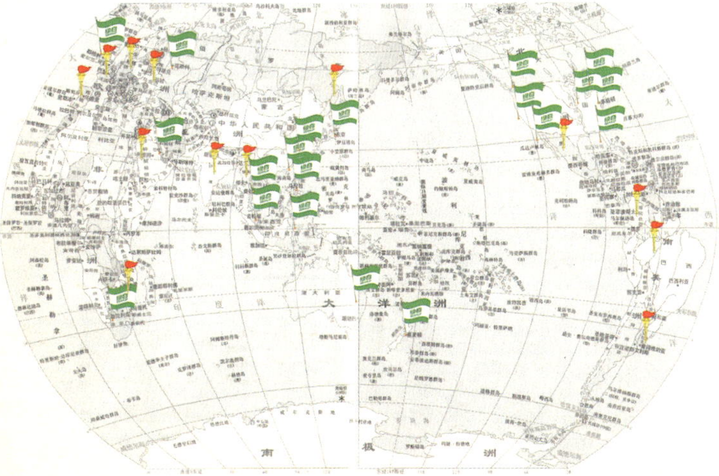

Green Valley Sales Offices (green flags) and Sales Penetration (red flags).

Additionally, this leading-edge company is currently developing specific formulas for many of the ailments that reishi has been used historically to treat. These include new products for hypertension (high blood pressure), diabetes, and immune-deficiency diseases. Great progress has already been made toward these goals. Additionally, the company has been conducting tests in South Africa on the efficacy of reishi powder as an immune enhancer for HIV/AIDS patients. Preliminary results are encouraging.

As a prominent Chinese company with many resources, Green Valley is well equipped to meet its goals and intends to do so using the highest quality manufacturing processes, as described in the next chapter.

Notes

Chapter Seven

China's Safety Standards

IT IS REASONABLE TO WONDER if SunRecome—a medicinal product manufactured in China—conforms to America's high safety standards. Here, the FDA diligently tests new medicines and carefully monitors reports of side effects. And the FDA does its job well. Of the more than 10,000 drugs approved by this U.S. federal agency between 1994 and 2004, only eight were withdrawn from the market for safety issues.[26] That is an impressive track record!

Can Americans rely on China's FDA for similar assurances?

Probably. Today's Chinese medical testing procedures are modeled after U.S. standards. Regardless, total reliance on the SFDA is not necessary, because:

- Reishi stands as one of the most widely researched and highly regarded herbs in the 2,500-year history of Traditional Chinese Medicine.
- Since reishi's discovery, there have been no reports of toxicity—even when it is used in large doses.
- Today's wealth of worldwide scientific literature validates reishi's historical claims of safety.
- SunRecome sales in China have steadily increased since 1997. These sales figures attest to the accuracy of the manufacturer's claim that SunRecome is a safe anti-tumor medicine:

SunRecome Sales (Converted to USD)		
Year	SALES REVENUE	% INCREASE
1997	$ 1.22 MILLION	-
1998	$ 7.30 MILLION	598%
1999	$ 24.39 MILLION	334%
2000	$ 38.18 MILLION	157%
2001	$ 52.12 MILLION	137%
2002	$ 63.03 MILLION	121%
2003	$ 85.37 MILLION	135%
2004	$ 134.00 MILLION	156%

- SunRecome is manufactured in a facility that is certified by the Chinese government for complying with Good Manufacturing Practices. GMP guidelines are established by the World Health Organization (WHO) to enable consistent manufacturing and quality control standards worldwide.[27]
- SunRecome's manufacturer complies with GMP standards by:
  1. Properly maintaining its equipment.
  2. Training its workers to perform specific tasks.
  3. Documenting manufacturing procedures so accurately that written reports can be relied upon to reproduce the product.
- Likely, the most impressive safety guarantee for SunRecome is the fact that this product complies with international standards for quality assurance and has earned the ISO 9001 2000 designation.[28]

What is ISO? Short for International Organization for Standardization, this non-governmental entity has become an international reference for quality management systems. More than 634,000 companies in 152 countries comply with ISO standards.

ISO 9001 2000 Quality System Requirements

SYSTEMIC REQUIREMENTS: establishing and documenting a quality system

MANAGEMENT REQUIREMENTS: supporting quality and satisfying customers; establishing a quality policy; carrying out quality planning; controlling the quality system; and performing management reviews

RESOURCE REQUIREMENTS: providing quality resources, quality personnel, a quality infrastructure, and a quality environment

REALIZATION REQUIREMENTS: controlling realization planning, customer processes, product development, purchasing functions, operational activities, and monitoring devices

REMEDIAL REQUIREMENTS: performing remedial processes; monitoring and measuring quality; controlling nonconforming products; analyzing quality information; and making quality improvements

Here are the manufacturing details revealing the quality systems under which SunRecome is produced:

Manufacturing Facility

SunRecome's multimillion-dollar, 215,000-square-foot manufacturing facility in Xi'an, China, contains the latest technology and boasts more than 20 different rooms, each devoted to a particular task within the production process. These safeguards achieve product potency and strict compliance with internationally recognized standards.

Personnel Management:

ADMINISTRATION ROOM: This staff training center enables each manufacturing and corporate employee to pass a test to become a certified reishi processor.

CHANGING ROOM: Each certified reishi processor that steps onto the manufacturing floor must first sterilize his hands, remove all personal items, then change into a sterilized clean-room jumpsuit. The employee's head must be covered in two layers of sterilized caps, and his feet must be wrapped in two layers of sterilized booties. Additionally, the changing room itself contains purified air.

QUALITY CONTROL: Supervisors maintain records on each SunRecome lot, including dates of production, raw materials used and quantities involved in the production process.

MONITORING ROOM: For quality assurance, banks of video systems help supervisors view the entire SunRecome production facility.

Environmental Control:

AIR ROOM: All SunRecome production rooms are fed by an air purification and filtration system. Five sets of air-conditioning units keep each room in the range of 64° to 79° F.

AIR COMPRESSOR ROOM: This massive equipment is designed to keep the air pressure consistent throughout the manufacturing facility.

CHILLERS AND HEATERS AND GAS BOILER ROOMS: High-quality equipment maintains the temperatures required by the various manufacturing rooms.

LOW-VOLTAGE ELECTRICITY ROOM: Sophisticated equipment converts the voltage for the wide variety of machinery involved in SunRecome production. This equipment comes from all over the world. Some devices require 220 volts, while others need 380 volts—China's high-voltage level.

WASTE-WATER TREATMENT: This takes place outside the SunRecome facility, in compliance with Chinese law and in line with responsible environmental protection.

Product Testing:

Please see Appendix 2 of this book.

LABORATORY ROOM: Experts regularly test for heavy metals in the water that is to be used in the processing of SunRecome. They also monitor the physical and chemical content of the product, the manufacturing facility's environmental conditions, and air quality.

MICROBE INSPECTION ROOM: Here scientists randomly sample each SunRecome batch to ensure against bacterial growth. Testing takes place three times: on the raw materials, after intermediate processing, and on the final product.

APPARATUS ROOM: Lab tests take place at every stage of SunRecome manufacturing. In the Apparatus Room, high-performance liquid chromatography (HPLC) testing and spectrophotometer recordings are emphasized.

SAMPLING ROOM: Laboratory personnel sample raw materials and inspect the finished SunRecome product.

Remediation:

MIXING ROOM: Reishi raw materials are mixed here, in accordance with the exacting SunRecome formula.

BUFFERING ROOM: Employees ensure that each batch of SunRecome matches the high standards of the original formula.

WATER PURIFYING ROOM: In this room, high-powered equipment is used to adjust water to the pH levels required for SunRecome manufacturing.

DRYING ROOM: Personnel dry the product after it is turned into a powder if its water content exceeds the established moisture-level standard.

GRANULE ROOM: SunRecome's powder is made consistently fine in this room.

Packaging and Storage:

SCALES: Each SunRecome packet contains 2 grams of the concentrated reishi extract. Employees in this room weigh each packet, number them using a computerized stamping machine, then place 15 packets into each product box.

ALUMINUM PACKAGING: SunRecome is double-sealed. The aluminum packaging machine automatically seals the product's internal packet.

COLD ROOM: This temperature-regulated room provides cold, dry storage of reishi raw materials, to ensure that they remain fresh, mold-free and medicinally potent.

STORAGE ROOM: This massive room holds the finished SunRecome product that is boxed and sealed.

Manufacturing Method

SunRecome's raw materials are also selected and processed with the utmost care, as follows:

Quality Fungus

Each batch of reishi mushrooms selected for use in SunRecome undergoes DNA analysis to determine its medicinal potency. And each reishi mushroom that is germinated in SunRecome laboratories hails from the highest quality "mother fungi" grown wild in the southern mountain ranges of China, one-and-a-half miles high, in a pristine area surrounded by streams and a valley.

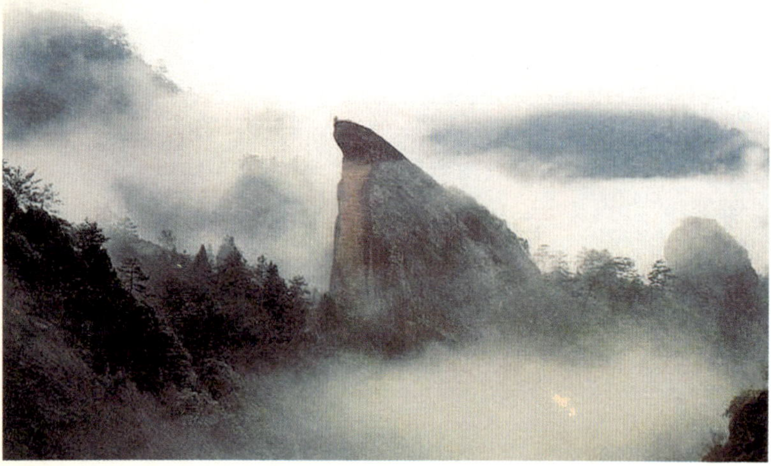

The Wuyi Mountains in southern China

These idyllic conditions provide the optimal soil and weather conditions to produce the best raw materials.

The spores from these potent mushrooms are grafted onto sterilized hardwood logs that have been drilled with 2½-inch-deep holes, so that reishi fruiting bodies can germinate through the wood. The wood logs are then planted in an environmentally controlled greenhouse that mimics the pesticide-free soil conditions, ideal seasonal temperatures, carbon dioxide levels, variations in light, plus moisture levels, high humidity and elevation found in reishi's natural environment.

Then begins a second generation of reishi, this time in an environmentally controlled laboratory created solely for the production of SunRecome. There, sterilized hardwood logs are inoculated with liquid reishi fungus, the drilled holes are sealed, and the logs are kept in a nonbacterial room. Before reishi mycelia penetrate through the wood, the logs are transferred to an environmentally controlled greenhouse.

Inside the greenhouse, mature reishi fruiting bodies will shed their spores, which are swabbed from beneath reishi's cap and collected in sterilized plastic film that is wrapped around the base of each mushroom's stem. Then the fruiting bodies are harvested, cleaned, dried and analyzed through DNA testing.

SunRecome Manufacturing Method

DNA analysis enables SunRecome scientists to extract the most potent active components from reishi's mature fruiting body and cap. Because many of these medicinal constituents are bound in reishi's hard, woody stalk, an ethanol alcohol and water extraction process is used to draw out the healing properties.

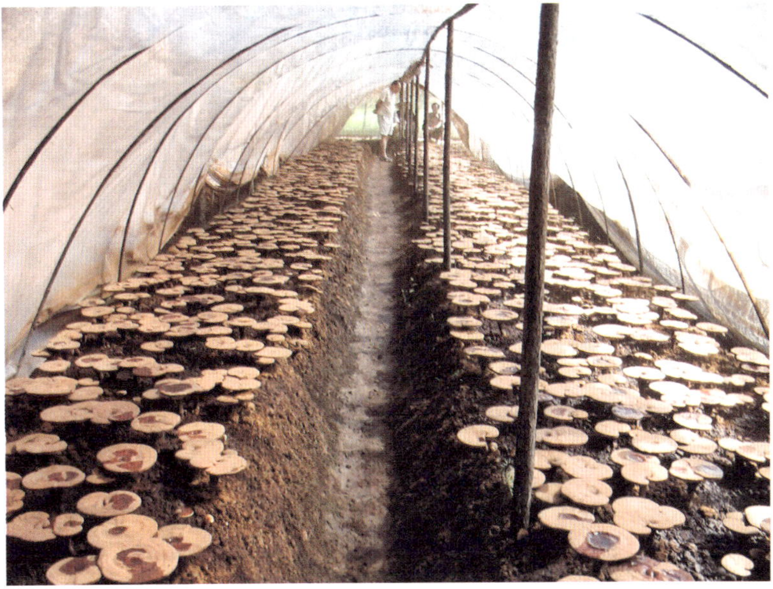

Green Valley's reishi greenhouse

Manufacturing consists of these steps:

1. Reishi's spore walls are broken via ultrasound, because these spores are coated in two layers of chitin—the hardest known natural substance in nature.[29]
2. Reishi's fruiting body is crushed into a crude powder and mixed with 60 percent ethanol alcohol.
3. The mixture is filtered, blended and condensed; the residue and remaining ethanol are removed.
4. Water is added to the residue to decoct the mixture, which is then blended, filtered and condensed.

5. The mixture and the residue are blended, diluted with water, and then mixed with the spores.
6. The resulting powder is uniformly mixed, sterilized and divided into 2-gram foil packets which are hermetically sealed at 149° to 158° F vacuum pressure to achieve a moisture content of less than three percent.
7. Packets are then placed in product boxes and sent to the storage room.

Hypoallergenic with Few Side-Effects

SunRecome is a highly concentrated extract. It takes 20 pounds of reishi's fruiting body to extract just one pound of reishi powder. And it takes 1,000 pounds of reishi's fruiting body to collect a single pound of spore powder.

So many people wonder how it is possible for such a highly concentrated product to be hypoallergenic and free of serious side effects. There is a relatively simple explanation:

Most allergic reactions are caused by proteins. During the extraction process, protein is removed from reishi. However, 1 in every 10,000 people will react to a pharmaceutically processed extract.

Individuals that do react to SunRecome report digestive upset or a skin rash, which may be evidence of detoxification. Such patients would benefit by taking a gradually increasing dose. Nevertheless, these reactions are quite minor as compared to the side effects from Western adjuvant drugs or radiochemotherapy treatments, which are:

Side Effects Reported from Western Cytoprotective (Cell-protective) Drugs

Abdominal or Shoulder Pain
Allergic Reactions
Anemia
Bone Pain
Changes in Mental Status
Diarrhea
Dizziness
Facial Swelling
Fatigue

Hair Thinning
Headache
Low Blood Pressure
Lowered Platelet Count—Increases the Risk of Bleeding
Lowered White Blood Cell Counts (WBC) — Increases the Risk of Infection
Nausea
Rapid Pulse
Ruptured Spleen
Seizures
Severe Rash
Sleep Disorders
Sweating
Tremors
Vomiting
Wheezing

Side Effects Reported From Radiochemotherapy

Confusion
Constipation
Depression
Dehydration
Diarrhea
Difficulty Moving
Fatigue
Fever
Hair Loss
Hiccups
Itching
Poor Appetite
Scars
Shortness of Breath
Skin Color Changes
Sleep Disorders
Sores
Swallowing Difficulty
Sweating

Swelling
Weight Changes

In human studies, SunRecome has not only been proven to be free of serious negative side effects but effective in strengthening the immune system during the onslaught of radiochemotherapy drugs. Now, for the first time, Americans can review these clinical trial results. Chapter 8 explains the testing procedures, while Appendix 1 of this book contains the unabridged SunRecome Clinical Trial Report.

Notes

Notes

Chapter Eight

The Landmark Clinical Trial

AMERICAN SCIENTISTS HAVE BEEN TOLD that no large-scale clinical trials have been performed on reishi. But the most potent reishi formulation available—SunRecome—has already been tested in the first two phases of a landmark Chinese clinical trial.

Phases 1 and 2, involving 160 cancer patients, took place from June to October 2000 in Xi'an, China, the former capital city. Trial results convinced the Chinese FDA to approve SunRecome as the first—and still the only—reishi formulation for use in conjunction with radiochemotherapy treatment.

Phase 3 began in September 2004 and will end in November 2005. Using both double-blind and negative control methods, this final round of testing will prove SunRecome's efficacy on an even larger scale than Phase 2. A total of 480 cancer patients are participating: 360 in the test group and 120 in the control group. Each of China's five most famous hospitals will test 96 cases to ensure the accuracy of findings.

Chinese law does not allow early release of official results and details. But the outcome of Phase 3 is expected to be consistent with previous tests and to reveal the effects of SunRecome on cancer of the breast, intestine, lung, and stomach, in addition to its ability to reduce toxicity. The clinical director characterizes the progress as "promising and inspiring."

All three testing phases were designed by the Chinese FDA (SFDA) in conformity with both United States FDA (USFDA) and World Health Organization (WHO) protocols, as applicable. Accordingly, SunRecome was exempted from Phase 1 testing, which determines safety, dosage, effect on the human body, and dosage form. When SunRecome was accepted for clinical testing, the SFDA was already satisfied that this 100-percent reishi formulation consisted of a time-tested traditional Chinese herb that is nontoxic in any dose, capable of boosting human immunity, and effective when administered orally as an extract.

Trial Participants

Phase 2 clinical trials determine the effectiveness (efficacy) of the investigational medicine (SunRecome) as compared to the control medicine (ZhenQi Fu Zheng Infusion; pronounced Jŭn-Che'Fö-Jŭng'). To make this determination, the SFDA requires clinical testing across a full spectrum of cancer cases. The Phase 2 clinical trial of SunRecome consisted of 160 tumor patients ranging in age from 18 to 65, both male and female. Patients suffered from a variety of cancers—esophageal, gastric, intestinal, liver, lung or mammary—in early, middle or late stages of progression. Though most were inpatients, some were well enough to participate on an outpatient basis.

All 160 patients served in one of four groups:

Therapy Group 1 received only SunRecome, the investigational medicine.

Therapy Group 2 received SunRecome in addition to chemotherapy, radiation or both, as appropriate.

Control Group 1 received only the control medicine, ZhenQi Fu Zheng Infusion.

Control Group 2 received only chemotherapy, radiation or both, as appropriate.

Control Medicine

In Phase 2 clinical testing, SunRecome was compared to ZhenQi Fu Zheng Infusion. Each product is described below.

Drug Resources:

Investigational Medicine: SunRecome

Produced by Xi'an Green Valley Pharmaceutical Co., Ltd. Batch Number: 20000301. Packaging: two grams per packet; 10 packets per box. *(Editor's Note: This product is now sold in 15 packets per box.)*

SunRecome contains the fruiting body, spore oils, triterpenoids and polysaccharides from reishi mushrooms (known in China as *lingzhi*; Latin name: *Ganoderma lucidum*). For more than 2,000 years, reishi has been classified as a Superior Herb because of its multitude of healing properties and record of safety. SunRecome, a concentrated reishi extract, has been used in China since 1997 to inhibit tumor cells, strengthen the immune system and minimize the toxic side effects of chemotherapy and radiation treatments. It is the only reishi extract approved by the Chinese FDA (SFDA) for use in conjunction with radiochemotherapy, and it is the most widely used adjuvant tumor therapy in China.

Control Medicine: ZhenQi Fu Zheng Infusion

Produced by GanSu Pharmaceutical Group. Batch Number: 20000107. Packaging: 15 grams per packet; 10 packets per box.

Zhen Qi Fu Zheng Infusion contains two herbs: Huang-Qi *(Astragalus membranaceus)*, a plant, and Nu Zheng Zi *(Ligustrum japonicum)*, a berry. These herbs have been used in China for centuries as a tonic to balance and tone the body, protect it from external disease, and enhance the immune system. Zhen Qi Fu Zheng Infusion, a concentrated extract from these two herbs, has been approved by the Chinese FDA since 1987 for use in conjunction with chemotherapy and radiation treatments to inhibit tumors and strengthen the immune system.

Here are additional details about the herbal blend:

Astragalus membranaceus: a native Chinese plant that has been used in Traditional Chinese Medicine for thousands of years. The immune-enhancing properties of this herb have been investigated in the United States for radiochemotherapy patients that are immunocompromised.

Much like reishi, *Astragalus* can help to heal a variety of other ailments, in addition to serving as an adjunct treatment for cancer. It can minimize or alleviate the symptoms of the common cold and flu, general digestive disorders, chronic hepatitis, high blood pressure, recurrent infections, lethargy and the physical effects of stress. It also has antiviral capabilities. Astragalus is a valuable medicinal herb imparting few, if any, side effects.[30]

Ligustrum japonicum: Relatively unknown in the U.S., this Chinese berry contains seeds that can stimulate the immune system. Ligustrum is under intensive scrutiny in China for its potential in preventing tumor formation and building human immunity. It is also used to treat fatigue, insomnia and poor appetite.

In China, *Astragalus* and *Ligustrum* are routinely used in fu zheng therapy, a Chinese technique invented in the 1960s when Western cancer therapies were introduced there and required mitigation of side effects.[31] "Fu zheng" means to fortify ("fu") and restore the basic functions ("zheng") of the body. Major Chinese studies concur that fu zheng therapy increases life expectancy for cancer patients.[32]

Aside from *Astragalus* and *Ligustrum*, other common fu zheng herbs are *Atractylodes*, *Codonopsis*, *Glycyrrhiza uralensis*, *Schizandra*—and *Ganoderma lucidum* (reishi mushroom)!

The fu zheng therapy compared against SunRecome in the clinical trial is a famous Chinese herbal tonic, ZhenQi Fu Zheng Infusion, used to restore *qi* (chē), which is vitality or energy lost during illness. In Traditional Chinese Medicine (TCM), when *qi* is exhausted, tumors can result because pathogens can accumulate. To improve *qi*, practitioners of TCM use herbal therapy, acupuncture, massage, *qigong* (a therapeutic exercise), and other techniques to increase a patient's immune function, life quality and prognosis.

Chinese Diagnostic Techniques

In SunRecome's Phase 2 clinical trial, TCM practitioners used tongue and pulse diagnosis to determine where *qi* was blocked in the trial participants.

Tongue Diagnosis

The shape, color and coating of a patient's tongue reveal that person's health. A healthy person has a pink and moist tongue with a thin coating that is either clear or white. An unhealthy person has a pale tongue, indicating a deficiency of *qi* or a blood deficiency, which is similar but not identical to the Western diagnosis of anemia. Other signs of imbalance or pathology include a tongue that is red, blue, purple, coated in yellow, coated thickly, scalloped, very dry or cracked.

Doctors of TCM help determine the location of illness through tongue diagnosis. Simplistically, the upper portion of the tongue reveals kidney and bladder problems; the middle identifies spleen or stomach ailments;

the lower third discloses lung or heart conditions; while the two sides pinpoint a disorder in either the left or right side of the liver or gallbladder.

Tongue diagnosis is a non-invasive, standard method of Chinese diagnostic investigation. Its results are cross-checked with pulse diagnosis to verify where *qi* is blocked.

Pulse Diagnosis

A highly skilled pulse reader can determine a patient's lifetime medical history and current quality of *qi*. This skill is honed by doctors of TCM through years of study and experience. From three positions and three depths of pressure applied to each wrist, these practitioners can distinguish 28 different characteristics of a patient's health.[33]

American Diagnostic Techniques

In addition to tongue and pulse analysis, the Phase 2 SunRecome clinical trial also incorporated Western methods of diagnosis.

Western-trained medical doctors confirmed the size and location of each patient's tumor via photographology, laboratory testing, cytology and pathology testing. Additionally, doctors monitored changes in patient blood values, immunology, body weight, urine, feces, liver and kidney function, and heart rhythms. All testing complied with diagnostic standards established by the appropriate Eastern or Western principles.

Research Methods

In the Phase 2 clinical trial, patient progress was deemed "excellent" if the ailment disappeared, life quality improved, and body weight increased; "good" if the ailment improved; and "no effect" if none of the above standards were reached.

Doctors verified improvements in patient health using internationally recognized statistical tests, called Chi-square, Ridit, and Adopt *t*-test. These parametric and non-parametric data measurements enabled researchers to make and verify assumptions about the extent that SunRecome can kill tumors, boost immunity, and stave off the negative side effects of radiochemotherapy.

The SFDA deemed the Phase 2 clinical trial results statistically valid (robust). The probability of error in these statistics is $P<0.05$, which means there is a 95 percent chance that the following test results are accurate:

Key Findings:

SunRecome is 85.7 percent effective when used in conjunction with radiochemotherapy – enabling cancer patients to complete their Western therapies and lay a solid foundation in the treatment of cancer.

SunRecome is 80 percent as effective as radiochemotherapy – giving patients that are ineligible for radiochemotherapy or surgery a treatment option.

SunRecome is 35.4 percent more effective than combination herbal therapy – proving that concentrated reishi alone outperforms the leading combination of medicinal herbs.

SunRecome is 20.8 percent more curative than combination herbal therapy – increasing the survival rate of cancer patients that use concentrated reishi rather than a combination of herbs.

Additional Findings:

SunRecome improves *qi* (vitality; energy) and blood quality by 88.57%.

SunRecome greatly improves dizziness and dim eyesight, fatigue and hypodynamia, hard breathing, insomnia, poor appetite, spiritlessness and lassitude, and spontaneous perspiration.

SunRecome can increase the tumor patient's body weight and life quality.

SunRecome significantly improves the abnormal physical signs of pale tongue and thready and weak pulse.

Additional Findings (continued)

SunRecome improves immune system functioning and peripheral hemograms, including NK cell activity, T cell subgroups, WBC counts, Hb counts and PC.

SunRecome is equally as effective on tumor patients of different ages and disease stages.

This clinical study did not include a sufficient number of cases to perform a statistical analysis on the effect of SunRecome on tumor size.

Patient observations did not reveal any adverse drug reactions or abnormal reactions on any patient's heart, liver or kidney.

Clinical Trial Director

The third phase of SunRecome's clinical trial is currently being conducted under the direction of Feng Wang, M.D. He is considered an expert in clinical trials, having spent nearly 20 years evaluating more than 50 clinical drugs for manufacturers and government entities. He has also published more than 100 academic papers on a variety of topics, including oncology, cardiovascular disease, hypertension, and anti-microbial agents.

Dr. Wang is responsible for preparing the SunRecome clinical trial reports. The entire Phase 2 Clinical Trial Report can be found in this book's Appendix. This report was translated from Mandarin Chinese to English in January 2005.

Notes

Chapter Nine

What's the Proper Dose?

IN CLINICAL STUDIES, SUNRECOME HAS been proven to enhance the effectiveness of radiochemotherapy and to minimize radiochemotherapy side effects better than China's most popular combination of medicinal herbs.

These same results are consistently reported by the doctors that supervise SunRecome patients in Green Valley's 15 service centers. They now offer detailed information about the proper dosage and other uses for this concentrated reishi formulation.

Preparation

Clinic doctors explain that SunRecome is consumed as a thickly concentrated mixture. Essentially, it is prepared much like instant coffee and looks a great deal like espresso.

Each individual serving requires water that is just short of boiling, ranging from 195° to 205° F. A single packet, which contains 2 grams of powder, is dissolved in ¼ cup (2 ounces) of hot water. Up to two packets may be consumed at one sitting. In that case, ¼ cup plus two tablespoons (3 ounces) of water are mixed with the two packets. The patient consumes the mixture when it is cooled.

SunRecome must be dissolved in hot water to release its concentrated triterpenoid molecules that suppress the growth of cancer enzymes in human DNA. That is why SunRecome is manufactured as a powdered extract rather than a more convenient encapsulated product.

Taste

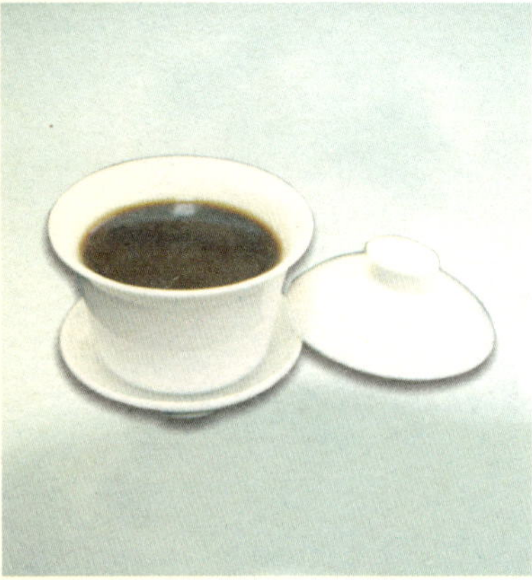

A cup of SunRecome

SunRecome tastes bad to the American palate, which is not accustomed to the bitter herbs that Chinese citizens have used as medicine for many millennia. And, unfortunately, SunRecome is especially bitter because of its key ingredient, concentrated triterpenes. Without this ingredient, SunRecome is the world's most powerful immune booster, but it cannot inhibit tumor growth.

So it would seem logical for Americans to add a sweetener to each SunRecome dose to make the product more palatable. However, clinic doctors strongly assert that adding any ingredient to SunRecome would render it 20 to 30 percent less effective. Additional ingredients, especially sugars, would be digested along with the SunRecome powdered extract, significantly affecting absorption of the product.

When pressed for advice, clinic doctors reveal that placing one tiny drop of honey on a patient's tongue before drinking the entire dose can reduce the bitter aftertaste. It is best to consume a cup of SunRecome in one or two gulps and to remember that the bitterness of this formulation is infinitely less objectionable than the side effects of radiochemotherapy or the continued growth of cancer.

Intervals

Just like many American medicines, SunRecome must be consumed on an empty stomach. For proper absorption, this product is taken no less than one hour prior to a meal or two hours after a meal. Patients that require two packets per day may take them upon rising and before going to bed. If more than two packets are needed each day, they can be added mid-morning and mid-afternoon. No more than two packets should be consumed in one dose for a maximum of four doses per day.

Dosage

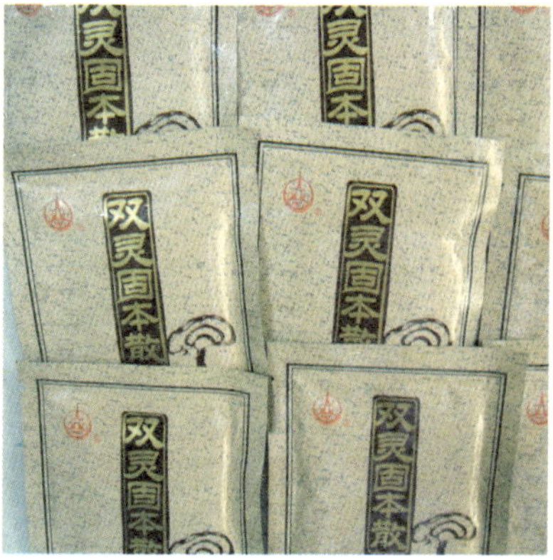

Packets of SunRecome

The proper dosage for SunRecome varies according to the patient's condition. Generally, newly diagnosed cancer patients take two to three packets each day. Those suffering from an ongoing bout with cancer take three to four packets per day. Late-stage cancer patients and those ineligible for radiochemotherapy take four to six packets per day. The maximum dose is eight packets, because SunRecome has no further effect beyond 16 grams.

Clinic doctors report that an occasional patient will experience some gastric upset or a skin rash at the beginning of SunRecome therapy. Some patients see dry, black stools, which is the color of the product, after the first dose. These generally mild side effects are evidence of detoxification. It is at the patient's option to work up to his maximum dose if the initial side effects are bothersome.

Course

A single course of SunRecome therapy lasts 45 days. Within 24 hours to 15 days, most patients report relief of chemotherapy side effects, including:

"Positive Side Effects" of SunRecome

- Cessation of vomiting
- Return of appetite
- Elimination of pain
- Good sleep
- Improved outlook on life
- Temporary immunity from colds and other viruses
- Feeling healthier than before cancer was diagnosed

After 45 days, laboratory tests can be performed to check for improvements in the white blood cell count (WBC) and other biomarkers specific to the patient's type of cancer.

Generally, newly diagnosed and medium-stage cancer patients use SunRecome for four to five months. Late-stage cancer patients and those not undergoing radiochemotherapy treatments benefit from taking SunRecome for eight to ten months. When there is no longer any active cancer, these patients can maintain their health with a half dose of SunRecome taken for 45 days. They can also consume an occasional packet to boost their immune system during the cold and flu season and at the beginning of a harsh winter or a rainy season.

Without Radiochemotherapy

SunRecome was developed for use in conjunction with radiochemotherapy treatments. However, some patients choose not to continue with Western therapies because they have experienced severe toxic side effects. Others choose to use only alternative treatments because they fear the long-term effects of radiochemotherapy. And many have no other choice because they are ineligible for radiochemotherapy: either they were already too debilitated when their cancer was first diagnosed, or they have become too weakened after having received Western therapies.

Rather than suffering through cancer without any treatment, SunRecome does provide these patients a viable option against the spread of cancer, as supported by the results of Phase 2 clinical studies. (Please see Chapter 8.)

Oral, Nose and Skin Cancers

SunRecome clinic doctors have developed techniques for treating certain cancers that would otherwise prevent the patient from consuming the product as a thickly concentrated liquid.

Oral Cancer

For example, some patients with oral cancer cannot swallow water. In these cases, the patient or an assistant can either mix one packet with hot water and use a dropper to administer the dose, or sprinkle the dry powder on the tongue for a day or two until water can be tolerated.

Nose Cancer

Patients with nose cancer can speed their healing by sniffing the dry powder through a drinking straw, in addition to consuming the liquid extract.

Skin Cancer

Skin cancer patients can mix the SunRecome powder in a small amount of hot water then rub the mixture into the affected area twice daily for 45 days. They can also consume the liquid extract for four to five months, or eight to ten months, depending on whether the patient is in early, middle or late-stage cancer.

Other Uses

For Radiochemotherapy Side Effects

For those most interested in mitigating radiochemotherapy side effects, SunRecome can be used just during these therapies. In these cases, the product is consumed beginning seven days before each round of treatment, and ending seven days after the round.

Children

Children can also use SunRecome. In Chinese herbal therapy, children are to take half the adult dose. Clinic doctors report good success at ½ dose for children aged seven and up and ¼ dose for three- to six-year-olds. Because the product has no toxic side effects, it cannot harm the growth of children.

Animals

In vitro studies proved that SunRecome is effective on cancer in laboratory animals. (Please see Chapter 5.) And the manufacturer is currently developing a product for veterinary use.

But at this time, SunRecome can still be used in its current formulation by dissolving one packet in ¼ cup of hot water then administering the liquid into the back of the animal's mouth via syringe. Exact dosage depends on the animal's weight. One packet is needed for every 40 pounds of animal weight, with a minimum of a half packet per day for 45 days.

Anti-aging

Although SunRecome was developed for cancer patients, it can be used in small doses for as long as desired to ward off the effects of aging. People aged 30 to 59 can use two packets per week, dividing each packet into three equal doses. It is important not to exceed this dosage so that the immune system does not become reliant on the product. Those 60 years old and older can benefit from using an entire packet daily, dividing it into two equal doses.

Prevention

SunRecome was not developed as a preventive therapy but for patients with active cancer. However, those who use tobacco, are physically inactive, have poor nutritional habits, are overweight, overexpose themselves to the sun, or skip routine health screenings can benefit from reishi capsules. When used consistently over time, this nutritional supplement provides immune-system enhancement via a four- to seven-percent concentration of the spore oils and fruiting body of the reishi mushroom. (Please see Chapter 5.) Reishi capsules do not contain concentrated triterpenes. For no less than three months, smokers should take nine to 12 capsules a day, two at a time on an empty stomach, while non-smokers should take six capsules a day. This nutritional supplement can be used indefinitely.

Best Effect

Some SunRecome clinicians believe that certain types of cancers respond better than others to the product. Because SunRecome was first used for digestive cancers, it is understandable that some believe this is its greatest application. They support this theory by the fact that SunRecome passes through the digestive tract. Other clinicians report the most frequent success with esophageal, ovarian, prostate and breast cancers. But the product's inventor, the manufacturer and the majority of clinicians refute these theories, stating that because the product boosts the entire immune system, it is effective against all types of cancers, even increasing survival time for leukemia patients. The Phase 2 clinical trial results support the majority opinion in that all types of cancers in the study—esophageal, gastric, liver, lung, mammary and intestinal—responded favorably to SunRecome.

Brain Cancer

Brain cancer is not as common in China as it is in the U.S. So it is important to report that SunRecome has been used the least on brain-cancer patients. Over time, it may still prove to be just as effective on brain tumors as it is on other types of cancers. In the meantime, SunRecome can at least help to mitigate the toxic side effects of radiochemotherapy for brain-tumor patients and extend their life beyond the oncologist's estimate.

Tumor Removal Theory

SunRecome's clinicians hold to a fascinating theory about tumor removal. Such removal requires surgery, which often leaves the patient with external scars plus internal scar tissue that can cause lesions and lifelong discomfort. That is why many Chinese clinicians believe that tumors should be rendered benign with SunRecome and radiochemotherapy but left in the body as long as they are not blocking vital organs. In Chinese medical theory, the purpose of cancer treatment is to attack the root of the cancer, treat its symptoms and prolong life. If it is not necessary to remove the tumor, Chinese doctors prefer to leave it in the body. SunRecome is reported to shrink tumors 50 percent of the time, to achieve some reduction in size 20 percent of the time, and to have no effect on tumor size 30 percent of the time. Former cancer patients that have used SunRecome successfully and now live with a benign tumor in their bodies do not report living in fear that the cancer will return.

SunRecome Clinics

In China, SunRecome is sold through 15 Green Valley service centers located in Shanghai and Beijing. These centers are manned by specialists in various cancers and herbal therapies. Staffing includes Western-trained medical doctors and doctors of Traditional Chinese Medicine, who all possess a lifetime of experience in hospital or clinic settings.

Chinese cancer patients learn about SunRecome service centers from corporate advertising in newspapers and TV, and from word-of-mouth. To date, more than one million cancer patients have used the product.

Cancer patients make an appointment to see a SunRecome service center doctor and bring a copy of their medical record. The SunRecome doctor reviews the history and performs a physical exam on the patient

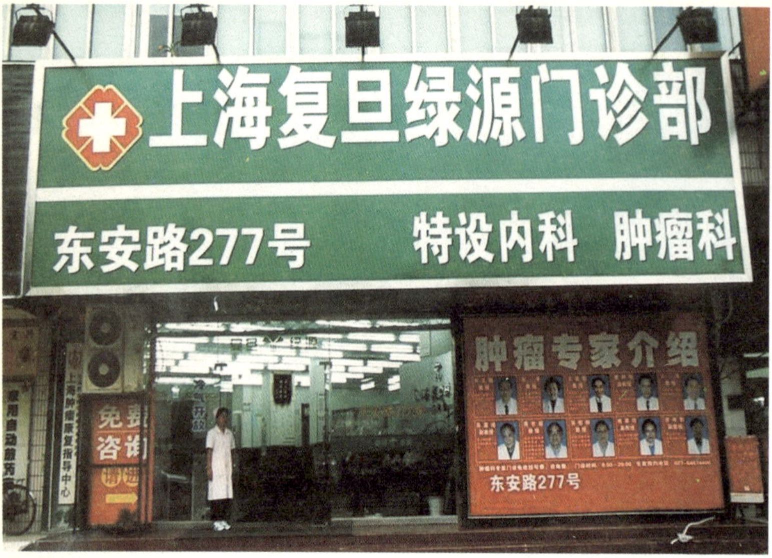

A SunRecome clinic

using both Western and Eastern diagnostic techniques. (Please see Chapter 8.) Then the doctor recommends a dose and course of SunRecome therapy that is specific to that patient's needs.

SunRecome service centers boast the best customer service for any medical treatment in the entire country. Without charge to the patient, each doctor supervises the progress of approximately 700 patients each year. Yet each patient receives personalized service, including weekly phone calls to the patient's home to check health status, unlimited in-clinic exams, and home visitation once a month—or more if the patient is unable to travel to the service center. Centers remain open 12 hours a day, seven days a week, from 8:30 a.m. to 8:30 p.m., with no less than seven doctors onsite at all times and as many as 20 doctors during peak hours.

Although it is unlikely for this model of customer service to be implemented in the U.S., it does explain how SunRecome doctors have become so knowledgeable about the details of each patient's progress, as reported in this chapter.

Cost

SunRecome is an expensive product. The average retail price for one box of 15 packets is $150. The product is costly for many reasons, including these:

- Only the best raw materials are used in the production of SunRecome. These are grown in a cultivation field that is located five hours from the manufacturing plant, by necessity, because of the exacting growing conditions that are required to produce a medicinally potent product. (Please see Chapter 7.)
- Purchase of the original capital equipment to manufacture SunRecome required an investment equivalent to $4.5 million USD, not including the cost of the 215,000-square-foot facility or its staffing.
- The manufacturer maintains a staff of 600 medical professionals to provide customer support in China.
- The USFDA clinical trial will cost tens of millions of dollars.

Despite the price, more than one million Chinese cancer patients have purchased SunRecome. Why? This product has been proven in clinical studies and in actual use to mitigate chemotherapy side effects and to improve the effectiveness of radiochemotherapy treatments in inhibiting tumors. It is considered the best adjuvant cancer therapy available today!

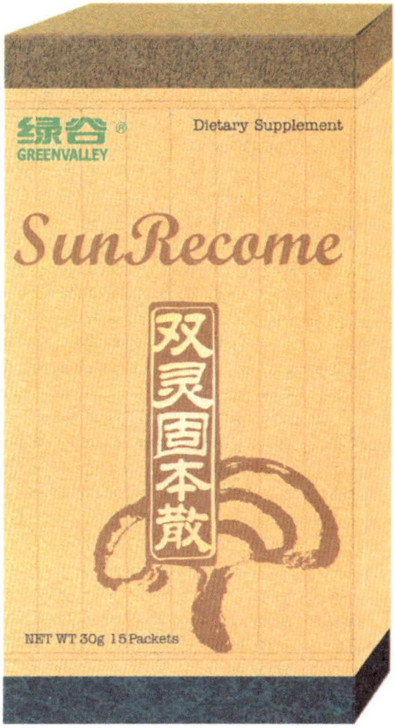

SunRecome box

Though the average household income of a Chinese family is roughly equivalent to $300 per month,[34] the price of SunRecome is not a deterrent. A typical course of SunRecome therapy lasts four months and requires three packets per day plus 45 additional days at half that dose for aftercare. The total treatment bill is in excess of $4,000, which exceeds the annual income of many Chinese! And the low maximum coverage of Chinese health insurance offers little assistance.

So to pay for SunRecome, most patients rely on the support of their family, friends and co-workers, who will give up everything to help with treatment costs. In China, these support systems are very strong and offer the best endorsement of this product's value.

Conversely, outside of public fund-raisers, it is unusual for U.S. cancer patients to receive much money for treatment from extended family, friends or co-workers. Instead, patients and their immediate families must shoulder the entire financial burden. But the U.S. Department of Health and Human Services (HUD) reports that the average American household income now totals $5,228 per month[35], which is a fortune to most Chinese. A bill of approximately $4,000 for SunRecome treatment is a substantial figure, but it does not constitute a fortune in America.

To explain their financial decision to spend more on SunRecome than they earn in a year, many Chinese cancer patients quote this well-known Chinese proverb:

> If the mountain remains, you will have wood to burn.

Roughly translated, these patients are saying that SunRecome can restore their health (the mountain) and give them a fresh opportunity to earn back the money (the wood) spent on the product. Americans might say, "Health is wealth."

In the next chapter of this book, several remarkable SunRecome cancer patients share their stories of hope.

Notes

Notes

Chapter Ten

Stories of Hope

More Americans Would Survive Cancer if they used SunRecome. This assertion is based not only on the SunRecome clinical trial report or the phenomenal sales record of this product, but also on real-life testimonies of patients who credit SunRecome for their survival.

39 Success Stories

Green Valley Fighting Cancer is the title of a 1999 Chinese book that contains the testimonies of 40 cancer patients who used SunRecome, 39 of which survived.

This book, written by Xue Ren Wang, a popular Chinese biographer, sold 10,000 copies. Most of the patients discussed in Mr. Wang's book had tried radiochemotherapy, while some had also tried surgery to survive their cancer. After all treatment options had been exhausted and these patients were in their final stages of cancer, they tried SunRecome—a relatively new product at the time.

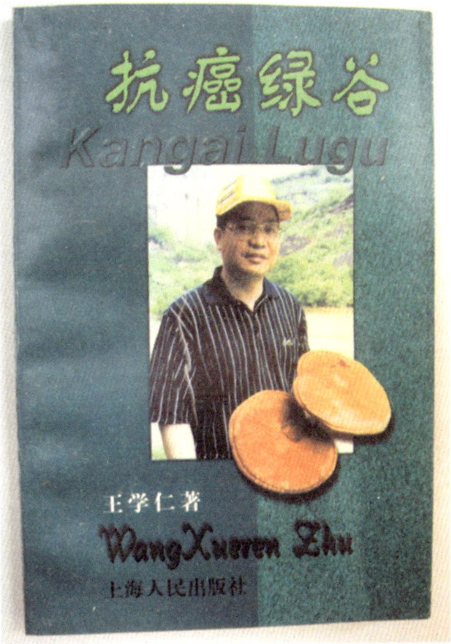

Book of SunRecome testimonials

All 40 patients reported significant improvements in their quality of life when SunRecome was used alongside their radiochemotherapy, including:

- Relief from vomiting and nausea
- Return of appetite
- Cessation of hair loss
- Increased energy
- Improved outlook on life

The 40th cancer patient described in *Green Valley Fighting Cancer* died one year after her course of therapy. Her ordeal was detailed in a second book by Mr. Xue Ren Wang, entitled *Angel*, which sold 8,000 copies.

The patient's name was Yang Ke, a young Chinese dancer. She began taking ballet and folk dancing lessons when she was just six years old. Her mother, a dance instructor, taught Yang Ke the importance of expressing inner beauty and presence while dancing. Under her mother's training, Yang Ke became famous and joined a prominent dance troop, which traveled throughout Asia to perform for state leaders. Yang Ke enjoyed good health and unusual stamina.

But in 1997, when Yang Ke was 14, she collapsed while competing in a sporting event at school. Her teacher discovered a swollen lymph node and rushed the child to the hospital. Tests revealed that she suffered from acute leukemia. She immediately began receiving full-body chemotherapy and became deathly ill from the side effects. News of her condition spread quickly via newspaper and TV accounts.

SunRecome's inventor, Dr. Jinshen Chen, visited Yang Ke in the hospital, and on behalf of the Green Valley Corporation, offered to donate as much SunRecome as necessary to help the little girl endure chemotherapy. Her parents gratefully accepted.

Yang Ke immediately began taking two packets per day of SunRecome and experienced no negative side effects throughout her 16-month chemotherapy treatment. In April 1999, Yang Ke's WBC count rose to normal levels. Soon afterward, Yang Ke returned to school and to her dance troop.

One year later, although she was healthy and strong, Yang Ke's Western-trained doctor recommended that the child undergo a bone marrow transplant to ensure that her cancer would not return. Her parents were

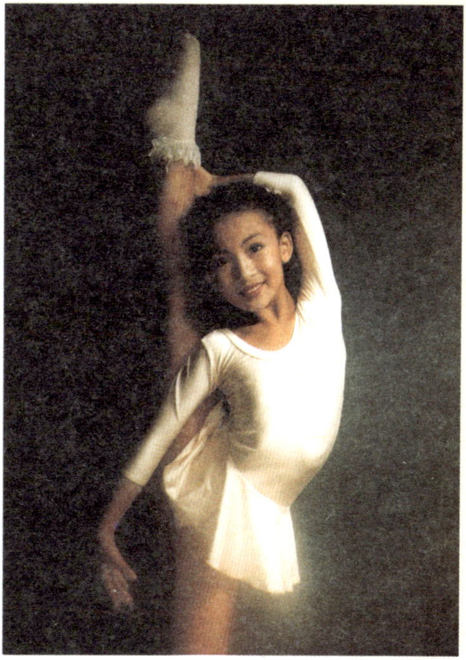
Ballerina Yang Ke

perplexed. Why would this doctor recommend such a dangerous operation when the child had been cancer-free for a year?

Yang Ke's parents consulted with Dr. Chen who agreed to meet with the Western-trained doctor. Dr. Chen, an M.D. himself, knew that standard Western protocol in leukemia cases dictates the need for a bone marrow transplant. Dr. Chen explained to the Western doctor that a transplant was not necessary, because SunRecome had already addressed the root cause of Yang Ke's cancer by starving her cancer cells, improving her immune system and repairing her damaged cells. Regardless of these facts, Yang Ke's doctor believed strongly in Western medical theory and continued to advocate the operation. The little girl's parents finally consented, not wanting to bear the burden of leaving any stone unturned to ensure the health of their only child.

To prepare for the transplant, Western doctors reduced Yang Ke's WBC to almost zero, which is standard protocol. The child suffered a great deal. To protect her liver, she was given a host of pills. Yang Ke chronicled her entire cancer battle and noted that she had been required to take as many as 80 prescription tablets in one day. Her liver function did stabilize, but her immune system had become so compromised that she developed pneumonia. Tragically, her Western doctor forbade the use of SunRecome to strengthen her immune system. The child's body began to reject the bone marrow transplant, and 300 days after her surgery, Yang Ke died.

Yang Ke's death shocked the nation. Her story serves as a reminder to stand firm when Western and Eastern medical theories clash. Green Valley doctors agree that Yang Ke would be alive today if she had not undergone transplant surgery.

Common Cancers

The good news is that more than one million patients have used SunRecome to date, and most have survived their cancer—all types of cancer. Meet just a few of these people who have suffered from some of the most common cancers found in America...and survived!

Lung Cancer

Major U.S. media and medical journals reference the website www.lungcanceronline.org as a leading source of lung cancer information. This site reports that: "Lung cancer is the number one cancer killer of both men and women and yet it is funded at vastly lower rates than the other common cancers. This has translated into fewer effective treatment options and an overwhelming 85% mortality rate." [36]

China's cancer solution—SunRecome—offers great hope for survival from lung cancer, as the following testimonial reveals.

Xingzhong Zhu, a former Communist Party secretary, smoked for more than 30 years before being diagnosed with lung cancer in January 2001. Before discovering the availability of SunRecome, he endured debilitating side effects from three rounds of chemotherapy, including weakness that caused him to be bedridden, in addition to excruciating pain and hair loss.

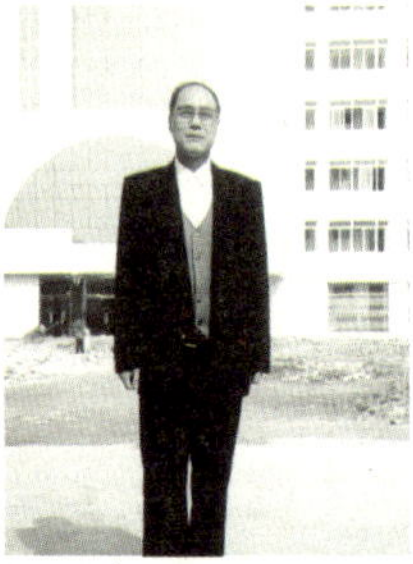

Mr. Zhu

Although chemotherapy treatments likely prevented Mr. Zhu's lung cancer from metastasizing, they did not stop the growth of his tumor, which increased from 2.1 cm. x 1.8 cm. to 3.9 x 4.1 cm. So Mr. Zhu sought alternative treatments, including a Japanese mushroom supplement and an experimental pharmaceutical for lung cancer. He was also examined by 42 medical doctors affiliated with the most notable hospitals in Xi'an. None offered Mr. Zhu any hope for survival.

Nevertheless, Mr. Zhu continued to search for help. He noticed a SunRecome ad in his evening paper and decided to attend a seminar that would explain the product's use in cancer therapy. The presentation included facts about lung cancer that closely related to his particular case. So, under the guidance of a doctor from a SunRecome service center, he began taking two packets of this product each day. After one week, laboratory results revealed that his WBC count had risen to 3,800. At that time, Mr. Zhu was strong enough to undergo radiation treatments to shrink his lung tumor. Within one week of combining radiation and SunRecome, Mr. Zhu's WBC count rose to 4,400.

But Mr. Zhu's treatment plan consisted of 30 rounds of radiation, which damaged his esophagus, resulting in a severe cough and an inability to eat or drink anything. The SunRecome service center doctor suggested that Mr. Zhu increase his dose to three packets per day. Mr. Zhu complied, and his ability to eat and drink quickly returned. Every three months, Mr. Zhu's WBC count was checked and it showed improvement each time. By the end of his radiation treatments, Mr. Zhu's WBC count normalized above 5,000 and his lung tumor was healed. In November 2002, he was given a clean bill of health but continued taking SunRecome for 45 more days. He also decided to give up smoking.

Prostate Cancer

The American Cancer Society estimates that more men will be diagnosed with prostate cancer this year than any other cancer.[37]

In March 2001, a woman's husband and her brother were both diagnosed with prostate cancer. But neither patient was told his diagnosis or prognosis.

Americans will find this common Chinese practice curious. In China, fearful patients are spared the facts about their poor health to prevent their fear from further debilitating them.

In these two cases, the woman, who was also a nurse, shouldered the responsibility for seeking medical advice and medication on behalf of her loved ones and for telling them they ailed from a less serious condition. Neither the husband nor the brother ever knew they had had cancer; thus these patients' names are omitted from this text. Additionally, some of the dates and diagnostic details are missing here. But the case can be substantiated through a newspaper article published on September 30, 2004 in the *XinMin Evening Paper*: *"regarding a Miss He."*

The husband's prostate cancer was severe: it had metastasized into his bones, liver and lungs. The brother's prostate cancer had not metastasized but the tumor was large and he was too weak to walk and could barely eat.

The husband was the first of the two to undergo radiochemotherapy and surgery. But these interventions had no positive effect on his cancer. Fearing the same outcome for her brother, the woman visited a SunRecome service center and purchased a three-month supply of the product.

She disguised SunRecome by placing the contents of the packets into individual bags used to dispense Traditional Chinese Medicines. Then she told her brother to use one bag of medicine a day, the equivalent of four SunRecome packets. On the tenth day, the brother was able to walk and his appetite had returned.

The woman was encouraged, and with the help of her children and younger sister, she purchased a three-month supply of SunRecome for her husband. He took the equivalent of three packets per day and soon after became eligible again for radiotherapy. After 30 rounds of radiation plus SunRecome use, his tumor cells were gone.

Meanwhile, the brother received a medical examination 20 days after beginning his use of SunRecome. This exam revealed a 1/3 decrease in the size of his prostate tumor—without radiochemotherapy. Moreover, in 30 days, his PSA index fell from 11 ng/mL to 3.7 ng/mL, which is within the normal range.

Both the brother and husband completed their SunRecome courses and still use the product during seasonal changes in temperature.

To this day, the woman is convinced that both her husband and brother would have died if they had not used SunRecome for their prostate cancers.

She firmly believes that it is the family's responsibility to seek complementary therapies for loved ones that are not responding to traditional treatments—even when medical doctors are unsupportive. She said that she would have felt ashamed if she had not tried everything to save the lives of her husband and brother.

Breast Cancer

The National Breast Cancer Foundation reports that "every 12 minutes a woman in America dies of breast cancer." [38]

In June 1998, Jian Fen Zhang was diagnosed with breast cancer that had metastasized to her lymph nodes. She underwent surgery to remove her left breast and surrounding lymph nodes. But the cancer had metastasized to her ovaries. She barely endured two rounds of chemotherapy before she could hardly breathe. And she was too weak to undergo another operation.

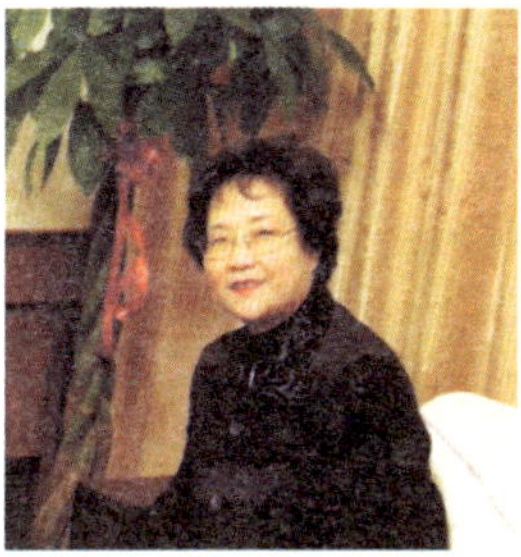

Mrs. Zhang, cancer survivor

During her hospital stay, she had befriended two other breast cancer patients who could not complete their course of therapy either, and had died. So when Mrs. Zhang's Western-trained doctors reported that she had no hope for survival, she lay in her hospital bed wailing for hours, convinced that "the demon of cancer would take her away from this world."

An outpatient from another hospital ward heard her cries and dropped in to see Mrs. Zhang. She shared that SunRecome had stopped her metastasis and renewed her strength, which made her eligible for radiochemotherapy to shrink her tumors. The woman cautioned Mrs. Zhang that the hospital's Western doctors would not be supportive of using this complementary therapy because they were unfamiliar with it.

Mrs. Zhang was skeptical of SunRecome's healing potential, yet she was determined to live. She phoned her husband who called a SunRecome service center for more information. That center sent a doctor to Mrs. Zhang's hospital bed.

Mr. and Mrs. Zhang wanted to try SunRecome but knew they could not afford it. So they purchased a small amount, and then sold their home to buy a six-month supply of the product, which she began taking at three packets a day. Within 45 days her strength returned and she became eligible for radiochemotherapy.

While using SunRecome, she simultaneously underwent chemotherapy plus 30 courses of radiation over a five-week period to her neck, breast and ovaries. Mrs. Zhang successfully completed these therapies without becoming debilitated!

Other patients in this hospital ward were not responding to radiochemotherapy alone and witnessed Mrs. Zhang's recovery. Before many of these patients died, they told Mrs. Zhang that they wished they had followed her advice to use SunRecome.

Mr. and Mrs. Zhang were fully convinced they had chosen the best combination of therapies available. Neither regretted the loss of their home to pay for the product. With her renewed health, Mrs. Zhang was able to take on a more responsible job, while her husband received a promotion that he credits to his renewed joy of life. Together they purchased an even nicer home than the one they had sold.

Pancreatic Cancer

The National Institutes of Health (NIH) reports that carcinoma of the pancreas has a markedly increased incidence over the past several decades and ranks as the fourth leading cause of cancer death in the United States. [39]

In 1996, Jinbiao Zhao was diagnosed with carcinoma of the pancreas too late to be eligible for surgery or radiochemotherapy. He lacked an appetite because the pancreas is an integral part of the digestive system. He also suffered from severe pain that woke him in the middle of the night, and from extreme lethargy. Doctors said his situation was hopeless. So this 49-year-old terminal cancer patient decided he would find his own survival solution.

He tried some alternative therapies, including shark cartilage and cordyceps capsules, to no avail. Then he happened upon a newspaper ad about SunRecome and wanted to give the product a try because he understood it could boost the immune system and inhibit tumors.

The SunRecome service center doctor recommended a dose of two packets per day, which Mr. Zhao purchased with the assistance of his family. In two days, his symptoms were improved: he desired liquids, and he was no longer waking up in pain in the middle of the night. In three days, he had enough energy to take a short walk. His general outlook on life was also improved.

In 15 days, Mr. Zhao was able to eat solid foods and to sleep continuously for five hours. His energy level had increased so much that he began to exercise each morning. He had the will to live.

After two months of using SunRecome consistently at two packets a day, he visited his doctor for an ultrasound examination. The results confirmed that his former 2 cm. pancreatic tumor was gone!

Mr. Zhao completed his course of SunRecome therapy and today takes two packets a day at the beginning of each season. He remains cancer-free, using no other herbal products.

Colon Cancer

Katie Couric, longtime host of NBC's "The Today Show," champions colon testing in memory of her late husband who died of colon cancer. Couric co-founded the Entertainment Industry Foundation's National Colorectal Cancer Research Alliance (EIF's NCCRA). This organization reports that "Colorectal cancer is the #2 cancer killer in the US; almost 57,000 Americans are expected to die from it this year. A majority of colorectal cancer deaths could be prevented if everyone age 50 or older were screened regularly, yet 41 million Americans who are candidates for screening have not been tested." [40]

Ping Li was diagnosed with late-stage colon cancer in August 2003. Doctors performed an operation that month, resulting in a fever of 104° that lasted for 11 days. When the fever broke, he underwent chemotherapy treatments that affected his nerves "like thousands of ants biting him from all directions." He could not keep food down and wanted to die.

Mr. Li's sister offered to buy some SunRecome for him, because she had successfully used the product during chemotherapy for breast cancer. Mr. Li had been amazed at the effect of SunRecome on his sister during chemo but was skeptical that this product could work so well for him. So he asked his Western-trained medical doctor for his opinion about SunRecome. The M.D. said, "If your sister wants to give it to you, take it. But don't buy it; it is very expensive and does not affect much."

Mr. Li accepted his sister's gift and immediately began taking three packets a day of SunRecome. During his second course of chemotherapy, Mr. Li reported fewer side effects. By the time his third round of chemotherapy was scheduled, he was feeling so well that his doctor allowed Mrs.

Li, a nurse, to administer the treatment at home. The treatment lasted from 4:30 a.m. to 2:00 p.m., yet Mr. Li reported being able to work for a few hours the very next day at his job as an activities director for a trade union.

When his health continued to improve, Mr. Li became overconfident, thinking that he could save money by discontinuing his SunRecome course of therapy for a couple of months. But, at this point, he felt much worse not using the product. After consulting with his SunRecome service center representative, he decided to reduce the dose from three packets a day to two. Mr. Li was tested cancer-free within a year of first using SunRecome.

Today Mr. Li is a remarkably healthy-looking man, who enjoys sharing his story of healing from a combination of SunRecome and Western therapies. More than once he has been challenged about ever having had cancer, because he looks so well. Eagerly he lifts his shirt for those who are skeptical to reveal a portion of the surgery scars that can be shown in public.

In Remission

SunRecome patients do not live in fear that their cancer will return, because they know that the root of their illness has been addressed. Their cancer has not been just cut out with surgery, or just radiated at the site of the tumor, or just subjected to chemotherapy drugs that kill the good cells along with the bad. Instead, SunRecome has increased their system-wide immune-fighting capabilities while attacking tumor growth, all the while maintaining the health of non-cancerous cells. Thus, these patients are not "in remission," as an American cancer-free patient is deemed, and there is no concern over one-year, three-year and five-year milestone markers. These patients are healed.

But anyone that ignores sound advice for staying cancer-free runs the risk of a cancer diagnosis. So in the final chapter of this book, five Chinese doctors mentioned in *China's Cancer Solution* offer their insights on how to avoid cancer.

Notes

Notes

Chapter Eleven

How to Avoid Cancer, Chinese Style

AMERICAN AND CHINESE DOCTORS AGREE that cancer can be prevented, outside of genetic influences, with:

- Diet
- Exercise
- Sun protection
- Abstinence from smoking
- Moderation in alcohol consumption
- Protection from infectious diseases
- Elimination of radiation and chemicals in the home and workplace

But the Chinese specify different foods and activities as helpful or hurtful. And they emphasize that attitude is of the utmost importance. Five learned Chinese doctors previously mentioned in this book now reveal the details about cancer prevention, Chinese style.

Dr. Jinshen Cheng

BEST KNOWN FOR: Inventing SunRecome

DEGREES: M.D. and doctor of TCM

BACKGROUND: Grandson of a country TCM doctor

"I think one of the main causes of cancer is an unbalanced diet. People who eat animal meat and fat will develop cancer more easily than vegetarians. Animal meats are acidic, and cancer cells can easily be born in acid. But vegetables and fruit are alkaline and contain the most vitamins and minerals. The best diet is 70 percent vegetarian and 30 percent meat. Specifically, try to avoid fried, pickled and salty foods. That will keep your body fluids balanced." (Please see Appendix 3 for a list of alkaline and acidic foods.)

Professor Zhi-Bin Lin

BEST KNOWN AS: "China's Father of Reishi Research"

DEGREES: M.D. and trained in Chinese Medicine

ASSOCIATIONS: Numerous. Please see Chapter 5.

BACKGROUND: Pharmacology and herbal medicine

"Learn to avoid or relieve stress, because it is toxic to your body. Exercise can help, as long as it is a fitness plan that you will follow regularly. Even a little walking or jogging relieves some stress. Do not stress your body from a poor diet. Avoid known carcinogenic foods, additives and drugs. For example, do not eat foods that are cooked at high temperatures, and avoid high-fat snacks, which we call 'foreign snacks.' Use healthful supplements, including reishi capsules, royal jelly, goji (also known as wolfberry fruit), *Tremella* (a fungus) and black edible fungus. These raise your immunity and can prevent many diseases, including cancer."

Professor Bing Xu

BEST KNOWN FOR: Inventing many chemotherapy drugs

DEGREES: Ph.D. in pharmacology

ASSOCIATIONS: Professor, Shanghai Institute of Materia Medica; Chairman, Chinese Society of Cancer Pharmacology and Chemotherapy; Director of the Shanghai Anti-Cancer Drug Consulting Center

BACKGROUND: Former visiting scientist in the schools of medicine at Columbia University and New York State University

"Lead a life that is free from smoking with little alcohol consumption. Do not drink stimulating beverages. Participate in sports but do not overexert yourself."

Professor Zhihong Li

BEST KNOWN FOR: Liver cancer expertise

DEGREES: M.D.

ASSOCIATIONS: Deputy Director of China's Anti-Cancer Integrative Medicine Committee

> "Increase your defenses with three types of immunity: psychological, nutritional, and physical. Always maintain a calm state of mind. Balance acidic foods with alkaline foods; take Vitamins C and E. Keep physically active."

Specific Exercises

The doctors referenced in this chapter are strong proponents of two types of physical activities for cancer prevention. These are called qigong (chē-gŭng') and tai chi (tī-chē').

Qigong, which means "cultivating energy," is a component of TCM that combines movement, meditation and controlled breathing. Qigong enhances the flow of energy (*qi*) in the body, improves blood circulation,

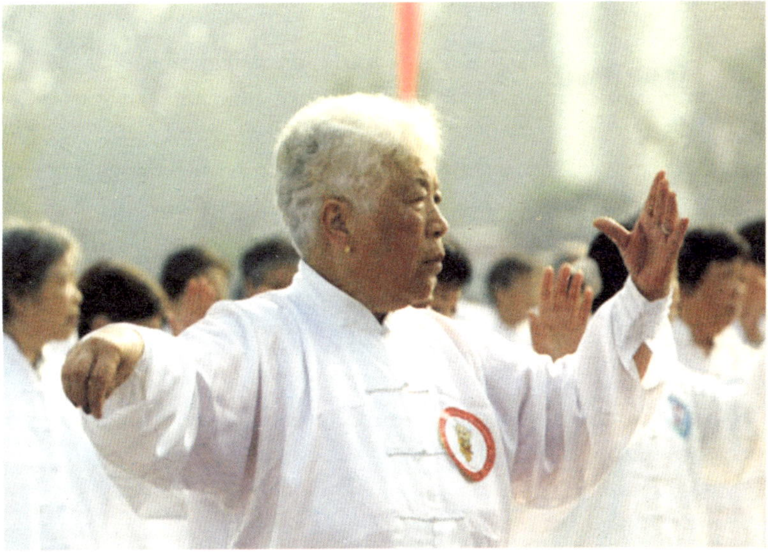

A qigong session

and increases immune system functioning. Qigong exercises are part of a national Chinese health-maintenance effort that promotes self-care. More than 20 million Chinese practice qigong daily!

Qigong is performed much like calisthenics and consists of six basic practices:

1. Stimulating acupuncture meridians to increase circulation
2. Directing energy to vital organs
3. Massaging the hands, feet and ears
4. Focusing on breathing techniques
5. Contracting and relaxing
6. Twisting the waist

Tai chi, which means "supreme, moving force," is a low-impact martial art that is also practiced by millions in China. Like qigong, tai chi releases blocked energy (*qi*). The exercises are performed as a dance consisting of soft, flowing movements.

The health benefits of tai chi include:

- Increasing the intake and sufficient use of oxygen;
- Reducing blood pressure;
- Increasing bone density by strengthening the legs, ankles, knees and hips;
- Expanding range of motion;
- Improving balance and coordination;
- Reducing stress;
- Improving immune system functioning.

Though there are many different styles of tai chi, their dance movements are similar and roughly consist of 13 exercises that begin slowly, warm to a quick pace, and then end slowly.

A wealth of data is available online about both qigong and tai chi, including exercise videos sold by:
www.amazon.com,
www.barnesandnoble.com,
www.borders.com,
and even www.eBay.com.

Professor Mingda Huang

BEST KNOWN FOR: Advancing the concept and practice of integrative medicine in China

DEGREES: Doctor of TCM; educated in Western medicine

ASSOCIATIONS: Executive Director of China's Science & Technology Cooperative Center of TCM

BACKGROUND: From a family of doctors who served China's state leaders; grandson of China's foremost expert in Western medicine

> "Anti-cancer capabilities exist inside everyone. Stay focused on self-regulation; never give up. Do not become angry; maintain a positive attitude. Exercise outdoors where there is fresh air. Prevent fatigue and cold. Eat anti-tumor foods, such as broccoli, cabbage and turnips. Consume sufficient nutrition: soy, eggs, milk and fish are the priorities. Take care of your whole body."

Professor Huang explains that to take care of the whole body, one must realize that while each body part has its own respective, important body function, all of the parts are interrelated and are influenced by the others. Disease occurs in a part of the body or in the whole body when there is an imbalance in the system.

In TCM, this imbalance is described as either Yin Syndrome or Yang Syndrome. Yin and Yang are polar opposites, resulting from an excess or deficiency in one or the other. This relative balance must be restored to overcome an illness, and the body must be strengthened to resist a recurrence. Treatment must be highly individualized according to the patient's age, sex, condition, locale, sensitivities and genetics, among other factors.

Whole-body balance serves as the cardinal principle behind China's system of medicine. This system evolved from practice and experience. While hunting for food, for example, the ancient Chinese realized that some foods could relieve or eliminate some diseases. While using fire for warmth, the Chinese found that applying hot stones or sand wrapped with leather or certain types of bark could relieve some diseases. While using stones as tools, they found that when a portion of the body is pierced, a disorder in another portion of the body can be relieved.

These discoveries became the origin and application of Traditional Chinese Medicine. Today, the TCM catalog includes more than 12,800 raw, medicinal herbs, in addition to healing techniques using heat, such as hot compresses and moxibustion, and the practice of acupuncture with its theory of meridians.

The Best Combination

Sometimes a person's best efforts at cancer prevention through exercise, diet, clean living and an upbeat attitude still result in cancer. The above doctors agree that if cancer does set in, the disease will affect all aspects of a patient's life: his physical, psychological, emotional, spiritual, environmental and social health. That is why doctors of TCM treat cancer as a disease of the entire body, even though it only manifests itself in one or more parts of the body. To help overcome it, TCM doctors do not rely on partial treatments, such as only chemotherapy or only radiation or only surgery. Partial methods do not address the root cause of the cancer— just its symptoms—leaving the patient vulnerable to a recurrence.

The doctors mentioned in this chapter cite the use of SunRecome plus radiochemotherapy as a prime example of a holistic approach to cancer treatment and an improvement over current cancer protocols through:

- Protection of healthy cells while starving tumor cells;
- An increase in the patient's immune system response while bombarding cancer cells with radiation or chemotherapy drugs;
- A significant reduction in side effects of radiochemotherapy, enabling patients to continue their Western cancer treatment plans;
- A new option for the survival of terminally ill cancer patients when they become ineligible for radiochemotherapy.

Using the best therapies that Western and Eastern medicine have to offer, patients will increase their chances of surviving cancer. And with more than one American dying of cancer every minute,[41] China's cancer solution comes none too soon.

Notes

Notes

Appendix

1. Clinical Trial Report

2. Supporting Documentation

3. Acidic and Alkaline Foods

PHASE 2 CLINICAL TRIAL REPORT OF SUNRECOME (formerly CGLE) FOR ADJUVANT TUMOR TREATMENT

(This report has been translated from Mandarin Chinese.)

Sponsored by:

Traditional Chinese Medicine Academy, Xi'an

First Hospital of Xi'an Transportation University, Xi'an

Traditional Chinese Medicine Institute, Xi'an

Shanghai Green Valley Holding Company, Ltd., Shanghai

Purpose:

According to Traditional Chinese Medicine (TCM), tumors are caused when qi (energy; vitality) is exhausted, which results in pathogenic accumulation. Modern medicine concurs that malignant tumors occur in combination with the decline in the body's protective functioning, particularly cell immunity, which enables tumors to grow. Such immune inhibition is most distinctive in advanced-stage cancer patients and in those undergoing chemotherapy or radiotherapy. Because a patient's immune function is closely related to his prognosis, it is necessary to increase immune function to fight pathogens. According to TCM, a patient's immune function, life quality and cancer prognosis can be enhanced by increasing qi. The purpose of this clinical trial is to compare the immune-enhancing abilities and safety of two well-known herbal extracts used in China for tumor therapy: SunRecome and ZhenQi Fu Zheng Infusion.

Summary:

This clinical trial consisted of 160 tumor patients observed from June to October 2000 in accordance with the clinical diagnostic standards for tumors. Patients represented a range in age, gender, symptoms, category, course and stage of disease, life quality, tongue complexion and pulse qualities.

Patients were divided into four groups, as follows:

Group 1, Therapy Group: Received SunRecome twice daily, one packet each time

Group 2, Control Group: Received ZhenQi Fu Zheng Infusion twice daily, one packet each time

Group 3, Therapy Group: Received chemotherapy or radiation therapy and SunRecome simultaneously, twice daily; one packet each time

Group 4, Control Group: Received chemotherapy or radiotherapy

Drug Resources:

Investigational Medicine: SunRecome

Produced by Xi'an Green Valley Pharmaceutical Co., Ltd. Batch Number: 20000301. Packaging: two grams per packet; 10 packets per box. *(Editor's Note: This product is now sold at 15 packets per box.)*

SunRecome contains the fruiting body, spore oils, triterpenoids and polysaccharides from reishi mushrooms (known in China as *lingzhi*; Latin name: *Ganoderma lucidum*). For more than 2,000 years, reishi has been classified as a Superior Herb because of its multitude of healing properties and record of safety. SunRecome, a concentrated reishi extract, has been used in China since 1997 to inhibit tumor cells, strengthen the immune system and minimize the toxic side effects of chemotherapy and radiation treatments. It is the only reishi extract approved by the Chinese FDA (SFDA) for use in conjunction with radiochemotherapy, and it is the most widely used adjuvant tumor therapy in China.

Control Medicine: ZhenQi Fu Zheng Infusion

Produced by GanSu Pharmaceutical Group. Batch Number: 20000107. Packaging: 15 grams per packet; 10 packets per box.

Zhen Qi Fu Zheng Infusion contains two herbs: Huang-Q (*Astragalus membranaceus*), a plant, and Nu Zheng Zi (*Ligustrum japonicum*), a berry. These herbs have been used in China for centuries as a tonic to balance and tone the body, protect it from external disease, and enhance the immune system. Zhen Qi Fu Zheng Infusion, a concentrated extract from these two herbs, has been approved by the Chinese FDA since 1987 for use in conjunction with chemotherapy and radiation treatments to inhibit tumors and strengthen the immune system.

Source of Cases:

Overall: 71% hospital inpatients and 29% outpatients. Groups One and Three: 71 inpatients and 29 outpatients. Groups Two and Four: 41 inpatients and 19 outpatients.

Tumor Confirmation:

Carcinoma in case study patients has been confirmed via photographology, laboratory testing, cytology and pathology testing.

Course of Treatment:

Thirty days in every group. Experimental subjects can receive symptomatic therapy and anti-infection therapy along with Western medicine, but they cannot receive Chinese or Western drugs for their therapy symptoms if they exhibit deficiency of qi and blood.

Research Methods

Polycenter, random, parallel and positive comparisons; positive comparison drug (control group): ZhenQi Fu Zheng Infusion

Cases Grouping and Trial Methods:

This trial complied with Open Label Trial Standards and abided by comparison and randomized principles. These standards require dose administration tracking by patient serial number and grouping; observation for any adverse reactions; cessation of dose administration if adverse reactions are observed; and reporting of any adverse side effects to clinical staff and trial sponsors.

Statistical Analysis:

- Comparison of measurement files: adopt *t*-test
- Comparison of enumeration data: adopt Chi-square test
- Comparison of rank data: adopt Ridit test

Diagnosis Standards:

- Directive Principle of New Chinese Medicine Used in Clinical Studies (M.O.H; P.R.C.): TCM
- Diagnostic Standards of Deficiency in Qi and Blood
- Chinese Diagnosis and Treatment Specifications for Common Malignant Tumors (M.O.H; P.R.C.)

Observation

Curative Effect Observation:

- Syndrome of TCM
- Life quality (scored according to Karnofsky Status)
- Immunology indexes
- Routine blood examination
- Body weight
- Size of tumor (measurable solid tumor: compared changes in tumor size)

Safety Observations:

- Routine examination of urine and feces
- Check of liver and kidney functions
- Electrocardiogram tests

Observation Methods:

- Syndromes of TCM
- Immunology indexes
- Life quality
- Body weight
- Liver and kidney functions
- Electrocardiogram
- Routine urine and feces are observed and recorded before the patient begins therapy and after three days after therapy is ended
- Routine blood testing is performed once before and once after therapy. Such testing is also reported in weeks 1, 2, 3 and 4.
- Solid tumor size is observed and recorded once before therapy begins and again four weeks after it ends.

Curative Effect

The total curative effect is determined in accordance with the Directive Principles of New Chinese Medicine Used in Clinical Studies.

Excellent Effect: Clinical syndrome disappears (or score values decline $\geqq 2/3$); life quality improves, body weight increases.

Good Effect: Clinical syndrome improves (or scores values decline ≧ 1/3); life quality becomes stable; body weight remains unchanged.

No Effect: None of the above standards are reached (or score values decline <1/3 than before therapy).

Life Quality:

Improved: Scores given after the therapy are ≧ 10 points more than before therapy.

Unchanged: Scores before and after therapy do not change more or less than 10 points.

Declined: Scores given after therapy are ≦ 10 points less than before therapy.

Immunity Reactions:

T-cell subgroup and NK-cell activity

Improvement: Immune function after therapy is increased or decreased by ≧ 10%.

Stability: Immune function after therapy is up or down by ≧ 10%.

No Effect: Immune function after therapy is decreased by ≧ 10% as compared to before therapy.

Body Weight:

Improvement: Body weight after therapy is at least 1kg. more than before therapy.

Stability: Body weight fluctuates no more or less than <1kg. before or after therapy.

Decline: Body weight after therapy is at least 1kg. less than before therapy.

Solid Tumor:

Complete Response: All visible focal disappears for at least four weeks.

Partial Response: Multiplying the largest transverse diameter and the largest vertical diameter of the tumor focal reveals shrinkage of more than 50% for no less than four weeks.

No Change: Multiplying the two diameters of the tumor focal reveals shrinkage less than 50% or enlargement no greater than 25%.

Progressive Disease: No new focal occurs but multiplication is increased more than 25%; or new focal occurs.

Safety Evaluation:

Lab testing indexes and clinical symptoms are evaluated in accordance with the Adverse Drug Reaction Report Monitoring Regulatory Method that was observed and analyzed for any adverse reactions in this clinical trial.

Adherence to Treatment:

This research team was comprised of trained physicians and nurses who dispensed medicines weekly and kept detailed records. Nurses supervised administration of medicine dispensed to both inpatients and outpatients.

Standards for Cessation of Trial:

Cases are ineffective if they are in accordance with items one, two or three, below; cases are eliminated if they are in accordance with items four, five or six, below:

- Serious adverse reactions are observed during the course of the clinical trial.
- Patients deteriorate and require critical intervention.
- Serious complications appear during the clinical trial.
- Patients cannot continue to receive treatment.
- Patients claim they entered the clinical trial for reasons other than a curative effect.
- Patients do not comply with the above standards; they do not take the prescribed dose; the curative effect cannot be determined; or incomplete medical files affect the conclusion.

Eligibility

Ages Eligible for Study: 18 to 65

Age Distribution of Group 1 (Therapy) and Group 2 (Control)

GROUP	No. of Cases	<31	31-	41-	51-
Group 1	70	2	3	15	24
	%	0.28	0.43	21.4	34.3
Group 2	30	1	3	7	6
	%	3.3	10.0	23.3	20.0

No significant difference between the first and second groups:
$X^2=1.304$, $P>0.05$ (by Chi-square test)

Age Distribution of Group 3 (Therapy) and Group 4 (Control)

GROUP	No. of Cases	<31	31-	41-	51-
Group 3	30	1	1	9	15
	%	3.3	3.3	30.0	50.0
Group 4	30	0	4	5	13
	%	0	13.3	16.7	43.3

No significant difference between the third and fourth groups:
$X^2=1.304$, $P>0.05$ (by Chi-square test)

Sex Distribution: Groups 1 and 2 totaled 100 people, with 45 male and 55 female = 0.82:1.

Sex Distribution of Group 1 (Therapy) and Group 2 (Control)

GROUP	No. Of Cases	Male	Female
Group 1	70	31	39
	%	44.3	55.7
Group 2	30	14	16
	%	46.7	53.3

No significant difference between the first and second groups:
$X^2=0.07$, $P>0.05$ (by Chi-square test)

Sex Distribution: Groups 3 and 4 totaled 60 people, with 37 male and 23 female = 1.61:1.

Sex Distribution of Group 3 (Therapy) and Group 4 (Control)

GROUP	No. of Cases	Male	Female
Group 3	30	18	12
	Percentage	60.0	40.0
Group 4	30	18	12
	Percentage	60.0	40.0

No significant difference between the third and fourth groups:
$X^2=0.00$, $P>0.05$ (by Chi-square test)

Disease Distribution: These calculations reflect preliminary data gathered from clinical symptoms.

Disease Distribution of Group 1 (Therapy) and Group 2 (Control)

GROUP	No. of Cases	<3 months	>3 months	>6 months	>12 months
Therapy Group	70	12	4	20	34
	Percentage	17.1	0.57	28.6	48.6
Control Group	30	3	5	3	19
	Percentage	10.0	16.7	10.0	63.3

No significant difference between the first and second groups:
$X^2=5.70$, $P>0.05$ (by Chi-square test)

Disease Distribution: These calculations reflect preliminary data gathered from clinical symptoms.

Disease Distribution of Group 3 (Therapy) and Group 4 (Control)

GROUP	No. of Cases	<3 months	>3 months	>6 months	>12 months
Therapy Group	30	6	7	6	11
	Percentage	20.0	23.3	20.0	36.7
Control Group	30	5	11	8	6
	Percentage	16.7	36.7	26.7	20.0

No significant difference between the third and fourth groups:
$X^2=5.70$, $P>0.05$ (by Chi-square test)

Disease Distribution of Group 1 (Therapy) and Group 2 (Control)

Disease Category	Therapy Group	Control Group
Esophageal cancer	6	3
Gastric cancer	9	5
Large intestine cancer	1	3
Liver cancer	9	1
Lung cancer	19	3
Mammary cancer	13	5
Other	5	13
Total	70	30

No significant difference between the first and second groups:
$X^2=11.28$, $P>0.05$ (by Chi-square test)

Disease Distribution of Group 3 (Therapy) and Group 4 (Control)

Disease Category	Therapy Group	Control Group
Esophageal cancer	11	5
Gastric cancer	1	2
Large intestine cancer	1	3
Liver cancer	0	0
Lung cancer	7	12
Mammary cancer	9	5
Other	1	3
Total	30	30

No significant difference between the third and fourth groups:
$X^2=5.34$, $P>0.05$ (by Chi-square test)

Stages of Disease of Group 1 (Therapy) and Group 2 (Control)

GROUP	No. of Cases	Stage I	Stage II	Stage III	Stage IV
Therapy Group	70	8	24	16	22
	%	11.4	34.3	22.9	31.4
Control Group	30	0	9	6	15
	%	0.0	30.0	20.0	50.0

No significant difference between the first and second groups:
$X^2=2.62$, $P>0.05$ (by Chi-square test)

Stages of Disease of Group 3 (Therapy) and Group 4 (Control)

GROUP	No. of Cases	Stage I	Stage II	Stage III	Stage IV
Therapy Group	30	0	15	8	7
	%	0.0	50.0	26.7	23.3
Control Group	30	1	9	8	12
	%	3.3	30.0	26.7	40.0

No significant difference between the third and fourth groups:
$X^2=3.82$, $P>0.05$ (by Chi-square test)

**Life Quality of Group 1 (Therapy)
and Group 2 (Control)**

GROUP	No. of Cases	60, 70	80	90
Therapy Group	70	47	19	4
	%	67.1	27.1	0.57
Control Group	30	24	6	0
	%	80.0	20.0	0.0

No significant difference between the first and second groups:
$X^2=0.09$, $P>0.05$ (by Chi-square test)

**Life Quality of Group 3 (Therapy)
and Group 4 (Control)**

GROUP	No. of Cases	60, 70	80	90	100
Therapy Group	30	7	11	1	1
	%	23.3	36.7	36.7	3.3
Control Group	30	0	14	14	2
	%	0.0	46.7	46.7	6.7

No significant difference between the third and fourth groups:
$X^2=8.09$, $P>0.05$ (by Chi-square test)

Symptoms

Inclusion Criteria:

These diagnostic standards for qi and blood deficiency in Traditional Chinese Medicine are in accordance with the Directive Principles of New Chinese Medicine for Clinical Studies (M.O.H, P.R.C). Patients included in this clinical trial had: a) more than three primary symptoms and more than two secondary symptoms simultaneously; or b) more than two primary symptoms and more than four secondary symptoms simultaneously (score of physical condition [Karnofsky Status] ≧ 60 points, anticipating survival duration > 3 months).

Primary Symptoms:

1. Fatigue and hypodynamia
2. Spiritlessness and lassitude
3. Pallid countenance

4. Dizziness and dim eyesight
5. Pale tongue with thin whitish coating and teeth marks
6. Faint pulse

Secondary Symptoms:

1. Hard breathing
2. Heart palpitations
3. Insomnia
4. Menstrual irregularity
5. Numb hands and feet
6. Poor appetite
7. Spontaneous perspiration

Exclusion Criteria:

1. People who do not exhibit the above symptoms.
2. People whose heart, liver, kidney function or hematopoeitic system is heavily damaged.
3. People who have a history of drug allergy.
4. Pregnant or lactating women; children; or psychotic patients.

Cases Eliminated:

1. Patients who quit the testing voluntarily.
2. Patients who disobeyed directions for taking SunRecome.
3. Patients whose potential response to SunRecome could not be determined or their medical files were lacking historical data.

Symptoms of Group 1 (Therapy) and Group 2 (Control)

Symptoms	Therapy Group (70)		Control Group (30)	
	No. of Cases	%	No. of Cases	%
Dizziness and dim eyesight	55	78.6	29	96.7
Fatigue and hypodynamia	70	100.0	30	100.0
Hard breathing	62	88.6	25	83.3
Heart palpitations	37	52.9	16	53.3
Insomnia	54	77.1	15	50.0
Menstrual irregularity	2	0.29	1	3.3
Numb hands and feet	12	17.1	3	10.0
Pallid countenance	69	98.6	30	100.0
Poor appetite	68	97.1	28	93.3
Spiritlessness and lassitude	69	98.6	30	100.0
Spontaneous perspiration	49	70.0	20	66.7

No significant difference between the first and second groups: $P>0.05$ (by Chi-square test)

Symptoms of Group 3 (Therapy) and Group 4 (Control)

Symptoms	Therapy Group (70)		Control Group (30)	
	No. of Cases	%	No. of Cases	%
Dizziness and dim eyesight	19	63.3	17	63.3
Fatigue and hypodynamia	30	100.0	29	96.7
Hard breathing	19	63.3	24	80.0
Heart palpitations	15	50.0	18	60.0
Insomnia	13	43.3	16	53.3
Menstrual irregularity	1	3.3	1	3.3
Numb hands and feet	1	3.3	5	16.7
Pallid countenance	17	63.3	21	70.0
Poor appetite	27	90.0	21	70.0
Spiritlessness and lassitude	21	70.0	27	90.0
Spontaneous perspiration	8	26.7	14	46.7

No significant difference between the third and fourth groups: $P>0.05$ (by Chi-square test)

Tongue Complexion of Group 1 (Therapy) and Group 2 (Control)

GROUP	Number of Cases	Abnormal Cases	Tongue Body		
			Corpulent and Pale Tongue with Teeth Marks	Corpulent and Pale Tongue	Pale Tongue
Therapy Group	70	70	13	38	19
	%	100.0	18.6	54.3	27.1
Control Group	30	29	8	17	4
	%	96.7	26.7	56.7	13.3

No significant difference between the first and second groups:
$X^2=1.15$, $P>0.05$ (by Chi-square test.)

Tongue Complexion of Group 3 (Therapy) and Group 4 (Control)

GROUP	Number of Cases	Abnormal Cases	Tongue Body		
			Corpulent and Pale Tongue with Tooth Marks	Corpulent and Pale Tongue	Pale Tongue
Therapy Group	30	19	0	7	12
	%	63.3	0.0	23.3	40.0
Control Group	30	12	0	1	11
	%	40.0	0.0	3.3	36.7

No significant difference between the third and fourth groups:
$P>0.05$ (by Chi-square test)

Pulse of Group 1 (Therapy) and Group 2 (Control)

GROUP	No. of Cases	Thready and Feeble or Weak Pulse	Thready and Weak Pulse	Thready Pulse	Moderate and Forceful Pulse
Therapy Group	70	12	33	25	0
	%	17.1	47.1	35.7	0.0
Control Group	30	7	18	4	1
	%	23.3	60.0	13.3	3.3

No significant difference between the first and second groups:
$X^2=3.51$, $P>0.05$ (by Chi-square test)

Pulse of Group 3 (Therapy) and Group 4 (Control)

GROUP	No. of Cases	Thready and Feeble or Weak Pulse	Thready and Weak Pulse	Thready Pulse	Moderate and Forceful Pulse
Therapy Group	30	0	2	18	10
	%	0	13.3	60	33.3
Control Group	30	0	1	6	13
	%	0	3.33	20	43.3

No significant difference between the third and fourth groups:
$P>0.05$ (by (Chi-square test)

Clinical Trial Results

Therapeutic Effect of Group 1 (Therapy) and Group 2 (Control) After Treatment

GROUP	No. of Cases	Total Therapeutic Effect			
		Excellent Effect	Good Effect	No Effect	Total Effectiveness Rate
Therapy Group	70	28	32	10	
	%	38.6	47.1	14.3	85.7
Control Group	30	2	17	11	
	%	6.67	56.7	36.7	63.3

Significant difference: u=2.74, $P<0.01$. Results show that the Therapy Group improved as compared to the Control Group.

Therapeutic Effect of Group 3 (Therapy) and Group 4 (Control) After Treatment

GROUP	No. of Cases	Total Therapeutic Effect			
		Excellent Effect	Good Effect	No Effect	Total Effectiveness Rate
Therapy Group	30	2	22	6	
	%	6.7	73.3	20.0	80.0
Control Group	30	1	10	19	
	%	3.33	33.33	63.33	36.67

Significant difference: u=2.89, $P<0.01$. Results show that the Therapy Group improved as compared to the Control Group.

Effectiveness and Curative Rates:

GROUP	PATIENTS	INTERVENTION	EFFECTIVENESS RATE	CURATIVE RATE
1	70	SunRecome	85.7%	88.57%
2	30	ZhenQi Fu Zheng Infusion	63.3%	73.33%
3	30	Radiotherapy, Chemotherapy, SunRecome	80.0%	93.3%
4	30	Radiotherapy, Chemotherapy	36.67%	40.0%

Life Quality Improvement:

GROUP	PATIENTS	INTERVENTION	IMPROVED	NO CHANGE	WORSE
1	70	SunRecome	58	5	7
2	30	ZhenQi Fu Zheng Infusion	14	14	2
3	30	Radiotherapy, Chemotherapy, SunRecome	7	23	0
4	30	Radiotherapy, Chemotherapy	1	28	1

Weight Changes:

GROUP	PATIENTS	INTERVENTION	INCREASED	NO CHANGE	DECREASED
1	70	SunRecome	49	14	7
2	30	ZhenQi Fu Zheng Infusion	7	19	4
3	30	Radiotherapy, Chemotherapy, SunRecome	9	16	5
4	30	Radiotherapy, Chemotherapy	3	23	4

Measurable Tumor Changes:

GROUP	PATIENTS	INTERVENTION	COMPLETE RESPONSE	PARTIAL RESPONSE	NO CHANGE	PRO-GRESSED
1	70	SunRecome	0	0	14	4
2	30	ZhenQi Fu Zheng Infusion	0	0	0	1
3	30	Radiotherapy, Chemotherapy, SunRecome	1	13	2	1
4	30	Radiotherapy, Chemotherapy	1	8	4	0

Symptom Changes of Group 1 (Therapy) and Group 2 (Control) After Treatment

Symptoms	Therapy Group (70)			Control Group (30)		
	Number of Cases	Effective Cases	Effective Rate	Number of Cases	Effective Cases	Effective Rate
Dizziness and dim eyesight	55	48	87.3	29	23	79.3
Fatigue and hypodynamia	70	65	92.2	30	25	83.3
Hard breathing	62	47	75.9	25	23	92.0
Heart palpitations	37	22	59.5	16	12	75.0
Insomnia	54	47	87.0	15	12	80.0
Menstrual irregularity	2	2	-	1	1	-
Numb hands and feet	12	9	-	3	2	-
Pallid countenance	69	53	76.8	30	23	76.3
Poor appetite	68	62	91.2	28	22	78.6
Spiritlessness and lassitude	69	64	92.8	30	25	83.3
Spontaneous perspiration	49	35	71.4	20	19	95.0

The Therapy Group's appetite improved as compared to the Control Group's: $P<0.05$. The other symptoms showed no statistical significance. No statistical analysis could be performed on menstrual irregularity and numb hands and feet, because the cases were so few.

Symptom Changes of Group 3 (Therapy) and Group 4 (Control) After Treatment

Symptoms	Therapy Group			Control Group			X^2	*P*
	No. of Cases	Effective Cases	Effective Rate	No. of Cases	Effective Cases	Effective Rate		
Dizziness and dim eyesight	19	14	74.7	17	10	58.8	0.35	>0.05
Fatigue and hypodynamia	30	23	76.7	29	14	48.3	5.08	<0.05
Hard breathing	19	12	63.2	24	13	54.2	0.35	>0.05
Heart palpitations	15	12	80.0	18	6	33.0	5.43	<0.05
Insomnia	13	10	77.0	16	5	31.3	4.30	<0.05
Menstrual irregularity	1	1	-	1	1	100.0	-	-
Numb hands and feet	1	1	-	85	2	40.0	-	-
Pallid countenance	17	9	53	21	9	42.9	0.09	>0.05
Poor appetite	27	23	85.2	21	17	81.0	0.15	>0.05
Spiritlessness and lassitude	21	16	76.2	27	11	40.7	6.03	<0.05
Spontaneous perspiration	8	6		14	5	35.7	1.77	>0.05

Results show that the Therapy Group improved as compared to the Control Group in regard to fatigue and hypodynamia, spiritlessness and lassitude, heart palpitations and insomnia: $P<.05$. No statistical analysis could be performed on menstrual irregularity and numb hands and feet, because the cases were so few.

Therapeutic Effect of TCM Syndrome of Group 1 (Therapy) and Group 2 (Control) After Treatment

Group	No. of Cases	Therapeutic Effect of TCM syndrome			
		Excellent Effect	Good Effect	No Effect	Total Effective Rate
Therapy Group	70	36	26	8	
	%	51.4	37.1	11.4	88.57
Control Group	30	5	17	8	
	%	16.7	63.3	26.7	73.3

Significant difference: u=3.25, $P<0.01$. Results show that the Therapy Group improved as compared to the Control Group.

Therapeutic Effect of TCM Syndrome of Group 3 (Therapy) and Group 4 (Control) After Treatment

Group	No. of Cases	Therapeutic Effect of TCM Syndrome			
		Excellent Effect	Good Effect	No Effect	Total Effective Rate
Therapy Group	30	16	12	2	
	%	53.33	40.0	6.7	93.3
Control Group	30	3	9	18	
	%	10.0	30.0	60.0	40.0

Significant difference: u=4.27, $P<0.01$. Results show that the Therapy Group improved as compared to the Control Group.

Tongue Complexion of Group 1 (Therapy) and Group 2 (Control) After Treatment

GROUP	Corpulent and Pale Tongue with Tooth Marks			Corpulent and Pale Tongue			Pale Tongue		
	No. of Cases	Effective Cases	Effective Rate	No. of Cases	Effective Cases	Effective Rate	No. of Cases	Effective Cases	Effective Rate
Therapy Group	13	13	100.0	38	33	86.8	19	13	68.4
Control Group	8	4	50.0	17	10	58.8	4	0	0.0

Results show that the Therapy Group improved as compared to the Control Group in regard to pale tongue: $P<0.05$.

Tongue Complexion of Group 3 (Therapy) and Group 4 (Control Group) After Treatment

Group	Corpulent and Pale Tongue with Tooth Marks			Corpulent and Pale Tongue			Pale Tongue		
	No. of Cases	Effective Cases	Effective Rate	No. of Cases	Effective Cases	Effective Rate	No. of Cases	Effective Cases	Effective Rate
Therapy Group	0	0	0.00	7	7	100.0	12	6	50.0
Control Group	0	0	0.00	1	0	0.00	11	3	27.3

Results show no significant differences between the two groups: $P>0.05$.

Pulse Manifestation of Group 1 (Therapy) and Group 2 (Control) After Treatment

GROUP	Thready and Feeble or Weak Pulse			Thready and Weak Pulse			Thready Pulse		
	No. of Cases	Effec-tive Cases	Effec-tive Rate	No. of Cases	Effec-tive Cases	Effec-tive Rate	No. of Cases	Effec-tive Cases	Effecti ve Rate
Therapy Group	12	12	100.0	33	28	84.8	25	4	16.0
Control Group	7	3	42.9	18	10	55.6	4	0	0.0

The results showed that the Therapy Group is better than the Control Group in regard to thready and weak pulse ($P<0.05$).

Pulse Manifestation of Group 3 (Therapy) and Group 4 (Control) After Treatment

GROUP	Thready and Feeble or Weak Pulse			Thready and Weak Pulse			Thready Pulse		
	No. of Cases	Effec-tive Cases	Effec-tive Rate	No. of Cases	Effec-tive Cases	Effec-tive Rate	No. of Cases	Effec-tive Cases	Effec-tive Rate
Therapy Group	0	0	0.00	2	1	50.0	18	9	50.0
Control Group	0	0	0.00	0	0	0.00	6	0	0.00

Results show no significant difference in pulse manifestation between the two groups ($P>0.05$).

**Life Quality of Group 1 (Therapy)
and Group 2 (Control) After Treatment**

GROUP	Number of Cases	Improvement	Stability	Decline
Therapy Group	70	58	5	7
	%	82.9	7.1	10.0
Control Group	30	14	14	2
	%	46.7	46.7	6.7

Results show significant life quality improvement in the Therapy Group as compared to the Control Group: u=2.91, $P<0.01$.

**Life Quality of Group 3 (Therapy)
and Group 4 (Control) After Treatment**

GROUP	Number of Cases	Improvement	Stability	Decline
Therapy Group	30	7	23	0
	%	23.3	76.7	0.00
Control Group	30	1	28	1
	%	0.3	93.3	0.3

Results show equal improvement in life quality between the two groups: u=1.51, $P>0.05$.

**Life Quality in Every Stage
in Group 1 (Therapy) and Group 2 (Control)**

Stage	Therapy Group			Control Group		
	Improvement	Stability	Decline	Improvement	Stability	Decline
I	7	1	0	0	0	0
II	21	1	2	4	5	0
III	14	1	1	4	1	1
IV	16	2	4	6	8	1

Stage I and II cases were combined. Results show that the Therapy Group is better than the Control Group in Stages I and II. By Chi-square test, Stage III results are: $X^2=2.037$, $P=0.36$; Stage IV results are: $X^2=3.915$, $P=0.141$. No significant difference in Stages III and IV between the first and second groups.

Life Quality in Every Stage in Group 3 (Therapy) and Group 4 (Control)

Stage	Therapy Group			Control Group		
	Improvement	Stability	Decline	Improvement	Stability	Decline
I	0	0	0	0	1	0
II	4	11	0	1	8	0
III	3	5	0	0	7	1
IV	1	6	0	0	12	0

Stage I and II cases were combined. By Fisher test: u=0.71. The result of Stage III is: u=1.57. The result of Stage IV is: u=0.52. No significant difference in any stage between the third and fourth groups.

Body Weight of Group 1 (Therapy) and Group 2 (Control)

GROUP	Number of Cases	Improvement	Stability	Decline
Therapy Group	70	51	11	8
	%	72.9	15.7	11.4
Control Group	30	7	19	4
	%	26.7	63.3	13.3

The results show body weight improvement in the Therapy Group as compared to the Control Group: u=2.55, $P<0.05$.

Body Weight of Group 3 (Therapy) and Group 4 (Control)

GROUP	Number of Cases	Improvement	Stability	Decline
Therapy Group	30	9	16	5
	%	30.0	53.3	16.7
Control Group	30	3	23	4
	%	10.0	76.7	13.3

No significant difference in body weight between Group 3 and Group 4: u=0.01, $P>0.05$.

Tumor Changes of Group 1 (Therapy) and Group 2 (Control)

GROUP	No. of Cases with Measurable Tumors	Complete Response	Partial Response	No Change	Progressive Disease
Therapy Group	18	0	0	14	4
Control Group	1	0	0	0	1

The low number of the cases did not provide enough data for a statistic analysis.

Tumor Changes of Group 3 (Therapy) and Group 4 (Control)

GROUP	No. of Cases with Measurable Tumors	Complete Response	Partial Response	No Change	Progressive Disease
Therapy Group	17	1	13	2	1
Control Group	13	1	8	4	0

No significant difference: $X^2=0.17$, $P>0.05$ (By Chi-square test)

Immune Response:

NK Cell Activity After Treatment (Immunofluorescence Test)

GROUP	Number of Cases	Before Treatment	After Treatment
Therapy Group	30	19.16±8.93	19.16±9.25
Control Group	30	21.84±4.79	21.03±3.57

No significant difference: $P>0.05$.

T Cell Subgroup Value Changes of Group 1 (Therapy) and Group 2 (Control) After Treatment

ITEM	Therapy Group (45)		Control Group (30)	
	Before Treatment	After Treatment	Before Treatment	After Treatment
CD_3^+	62.44±3.61	69.72±5.76	62.27±3.97	62.97±4.02
CD_4^+	40.01±4.32	45.36±5.09	42.33±2.36	41.96±2.72
CD_8^+	22.90±2.65	27.62±2.92	22.77±2.03	22.79±2.05

By t test, CD_3^+ ,CD_4^+ and CD_8^+ improved in the Therapy Group after treatment. The Therapy Group was better than the Control Group in CD_3^+, CD_4^+ and CD_8^+ after treatment.

T Cell Subgroup Value Changes of Group 3 (Therapy) and Group 4 (Control) After Treatment

ITEM	Therapy Group (30)		Control Group (30)	
	Before Treatment	After Treatment	Before Treatment	After Treatment
CD3+	59.91±12.49	57.48±10.03	59.37±11.6	58.7±9.82
CD4+	33.74±9.18	35.26±8.91	37.10±11.72	36.47±8.10
CD8+	25.68±7.59	25.08±7.78	23.1±5.65	22.45±5.05

By t test, there is no significant difference between the two groups in CD_3^+, CD_4^+ and CD_8^+ after treatment.

Ratio of CD_4^+ to CD_8^+ of Group 1 (Therapy) and Group 2 (Control) After Treatment (x ±SD)

GROUP	Number of Cases	Before Treatment	After Treatment
Therapy Group	45	1.76±0.22	1.65±0.17
Control Group	30	1.864±0.128	1.85±0.11

Results show that CD_4^+ / CD_8^+have significant differences in the Therapy Group before and after treatment: t=2.65, $P<0.01$. The Therapy Group was better than the Control Group in the ratio of CD_4^+ / CD_8^+: t=5.69, $P<0.01$.

Ratio of CD_4^+ to CD_8^+ of Group 3 (Therapy) and Group 4 (Control) After Treatment (x ±SD)

GROUP	Number of Cases	Before Treatment	After Treatment
Therapy Group	30	1.46±0.66	1.57±0.77
Control Group	30	1.66±0.51	1.69±0.51

No significant difference: t=0.61, $P>0.05$.

Peripheral Hemogram:

White Blood Cell Changes of Group 1 (Therapy) and Group 2 (Control) After Treatment (x ±SD, 10^9/L)

GROUP	Abnormal Cases	Before Treatment	Value Difference
Therapy Group	23	2.94±0.76	1.67±1.85
Control Group	11	2.98±0.53	3.01±1.86

WBC count is increased after treatment in the Therapy Group (t=4.30, $P<0.01$). There was no significant difference between the two groups after treatment: $P>0.05$.

White Blood Cell Changes of Group 3 (Therapy) and Group 4 (Control) After Treatment (x ±SD, 10^9/L)

GROUP	Abnormal Cases	Before Treatment	Value Difference
Therapy Group	16	3.03±0.76	2.36±2.30
Control Group	8	3.36±0.40	1.80±1.04

WBC count was increased after treatment in Therapy Group (t=4.10, $P<0.01$). There was no significant difference between the two groups after treatment ($P>0.05$).

Hemoglobin Changes in
Group 1 (Therapy) and Group 2 (Control) (x ±SD, g/L)

GROUP	Abnormal Cases	Before Treatment	Value Difference
Therapy Group	27	94.52±16.21	16.96±25.50
Control Group	10	87.70±11.25	27.70±19.75

Hb increased in the Therapy Group after treatment: t=3.44, $P<0.01$. There was no other significant difference between the two groups after treatment ($P>0.05$).

Hemoglobin Changes in
Group 3 (Therapy) and Group 4 (Control)
After Treatment (□±SD, g/L)

GROUP	Abnormal Cases	Before Treatment	Value Difference
Therapy Group	17	102.9±10.27	6.12±8.64
Control Group	16	102.19±12.23	7.31±12.44

Hb increased in the Therapy Group after treatment: t=2.92, $P<0.01$. There was no other significant difference between the two groups after treatment: $P>0.05$.

Platelet Changes in
Group 1 (Therapy) and Group 2 (Control)
After Treatment (x ±SD, 109/L)

GROUP	Abnormal Cases	Before Treatment	Value Difference
Therapy Group	28	66.3±19.1	41.39±48.25
Control Group	14	61.29±25.28	50.00±38.28

PC count increased in the Therapy Group after treatment: t=4.46, $P<0.01$. There was no other significant difference between the two groups after treatment: $P>0.05$.

Platelet Changes in Group 3 (Therapy) and Group 4 (Control) After Treatment (x ±SD, 10^9/L)

GROUP	Abnormal Cases	Before Treatment	Value Difference
Therapy Group	8	83.88±11.12	56.13±63.92
Control Group	4	88.50±11.84	23.50±12.70

PC count increased in the Therapy Group after treatment: t=2.48, $P<0.01$. There was no other significant difference between the two groups after treatment: $P>0.05$.

Comparison of Age and the Curative Effect in Group 1 (Therapy) and Group 2 (Control Group)

Age	Curative Effect		
	Excellent Effect	Good Effect	No Effect
<31	1	1	0
31-	2	1	0
41-	4	6	5
51-	11	10	3
61-65	10	14	2

No significance in the Therapy Group: u=1.41, $P>0.05$.

Comparison of Age and the Curative Effect in Group 3 (Therapy) and Group 4 (Control)

Age	Curative Effect		
	Excellent Effect	Good Effect	No Effect
<31	0	1	0
31-	0	1	0
41-	0	7	2
51-	2	10	3
61-65	0	3	1

No significance in the Therapy Group: u=0.40, $P>0.05$.

Disease Category and the Curative Effect in Group 1 (Therapy) and Group 2 (Control)

Disease Category	Curative Effect		
	Excellent Effect	Good Effect	No Effect
Esophageal Cancer	1	4	1
Gastric Cancer	4	2	3
Liver Cancer	2	4	3
Lung Cancer	8	11	0
Mammary Cancer	6	5	2
Intestinal Cancer	4	5	0
Other	3	1	1

No significance in the Therapy Group: u=0.59, $P>0.05$.

Disease Category and the Curative Effect in Group 3 (Therapy) and Group 4 (Control)

Disease Category	Curative Effect		
	Excellent Effect	Good Effect	No Effect
Lung Cancer	0	4	3
Gastric Cancer	1	0	0
Liver Cancer	0	0	0
Mammary Cancer	0	8	1
Esophageal Cancer	1	8	2
Intestinal Cancer	0	1	0
Other	0	1	0

No significance in the Therapy Group: u=1.60, $P>0.05$.

Evaluation of Adverse Reactions

The Therapy Groups did not experience any toxic effects, side effects or adverse reactions from SunRecome.

Analysis of Eliminated and Lost Cases

One patient died of exacerbation, one was out of contact in the Therapy Group, and one was out of contact with the hospital in the Control Group.

Evaluation of Adherence to Treatment

All cases had good adherence to treatment in the Therapy Groups.

Conclusions

Statistical analysis of this clinical study reveals that the Therapy Groups improved as compared to the Control Groups. SunRecome offered Therapy Group patients a good adjuvant curative effect, regardless of the patient's age, gender, disease category or stage of illness. Additionally, Therapy Group patients increased in life quality and body weight. Immune system analysis showed that NK cell activity significantly improved in the Therapy Groups as compared to the Control Groups. Patient observation did not reveal any abnormal alteration to heart, liver or kidney. There were no adverse reactions resulting from the administration of SunRecome.

Findings:

1. SunRecome is 85.7% effective when used in conjunction with radiochemotherapy.
2. SunRecome is 80% as effective as radiochemotherapy.
3. SunRecome is 35.4% more effective and 20.8% more curative than ZhenQi Fu Zheng Infusion.
4. SunRecome improves qi (vitality; energy) and blood quality by 88.57%.
5. SunRecome greatly improves dizziness and dim eyesight, fatigue and hypodynamia, hard breathing, insomnia, poor appetite, spiritlessness and lassitude, and spontaneous perspiration.
6. SunRecome can increase the tumor patient's body weight and life quality.

7. SunRecome significantly improves the abnormal physical signs of pale tongue and thready and weak pulse.
8. SunRecome improves immune system functioning and peripheral hemograms, including NK cell activity, T cell subgroups, WBC counts, Hb counts and PC.
9. SunRecome is equally as effective on tumor patients of different ages and disease stages.
10. This clinical study did not include a sufficient number of cases to perform a statistical analysis on the effect of SunRecome on tumor size.
11. Patient observations did not reveal any adverse drug reactions or abnormal reactions on any patient's heart, liver or kidney.

APPENDIX 2
Supporting Documentation

SUNRECOME PATENT AWARD

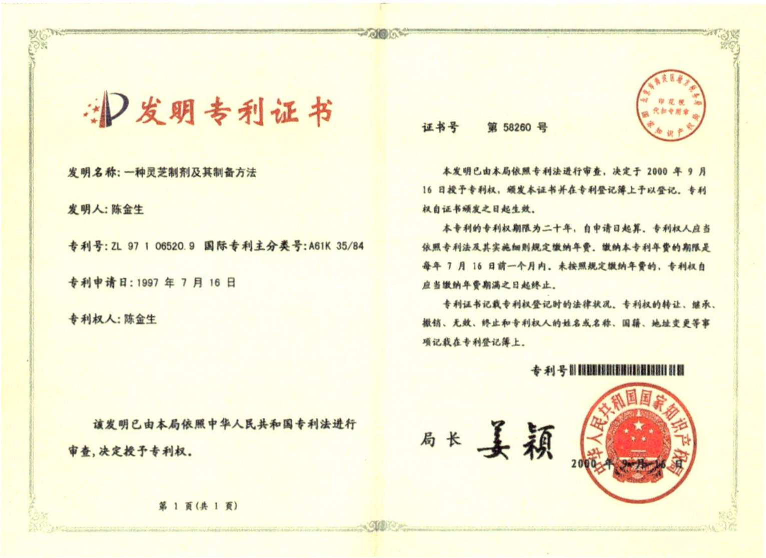

发明专利证书

发明名称: 一种灵芝制剂及其制备方法

发明人: 陈金生

专利号: ZL 97 1 06520.9 国际专利主分类号: A61K 35/84

专利申请日: 1997 年 7 月 16 日

专利权人: 陈金生

该发明已由本局依照中华人民共和国专利法进行审查, 决定授予专利权。

第 1 页(共 1 页)

证书号 第 58260 号

本发明已由本局依照专利法进行审查, 决定于 2000 年 9 月 16 日授予专利权, 颁发本证书并在专利登记簿上予以登记。专利权自证书颁发之日起生效。

本专利的专利权期限为二十年, 自申请日起算。专利权人应当依照专利法及其实施细则规定缴纳年费。缴纳本专利年费的期限是每年 7 月 16 日前一个月内。未按照规定缴纳年费的, 专利权自应当缴纳年费期满之日起终止。

专利证书记载专利权登记时的法律状况。专利权的转让、继承、撤销、无效、终止和专利权人的姓名或名称、国籍、地址变更等事项记载在专利登记簿上。

专利号

局长 姜颖

2000 年 9 月 16 日

SFDA CERTIFICATE

国家药品监督管理局批件

受理号：BZ1615　　　　批件号：2002B0798

药品名称	中文名称：双灵固本散 汉语拼音：Shuangling Guben San		
剂　　型	散剂	规　　格	每袋装2g
生产企业	西安绿谷制药有限公司		
生产地址	西安市丈八东路2号		
初审单位	陕西省药品监督管理局		
审批结论	同意生产，并核发药品批准文号，注销原批准文号。 在标准试行期间，继续积累本品的含测数据，考察本品的稳定性。		
药品批准文号	国药准字B20020428	原批准文号	陕卫药健字(1996)第0101号
附　　件	质量标准、说明书及标签	标准编号	WS-5407(B-0407)-2002
主　　送	陕西省药品监督管理局		
抄　　送	陕西省药品检验所，中国药品生物制品检定所，国家药典委员会，国家药品监督管理局药品审评中心，西安绿谷制药有限公司，药品安全监管司、市场监督司		
备　　注	本批件及其所附质量标准、说明书及标签自2002年11月28日起生效。		

CERTIFICATE AWARDED TO GV AS A
TOP 100 PRIVATE HIGH-TECH ENTERPRISE IN SHANGHAI

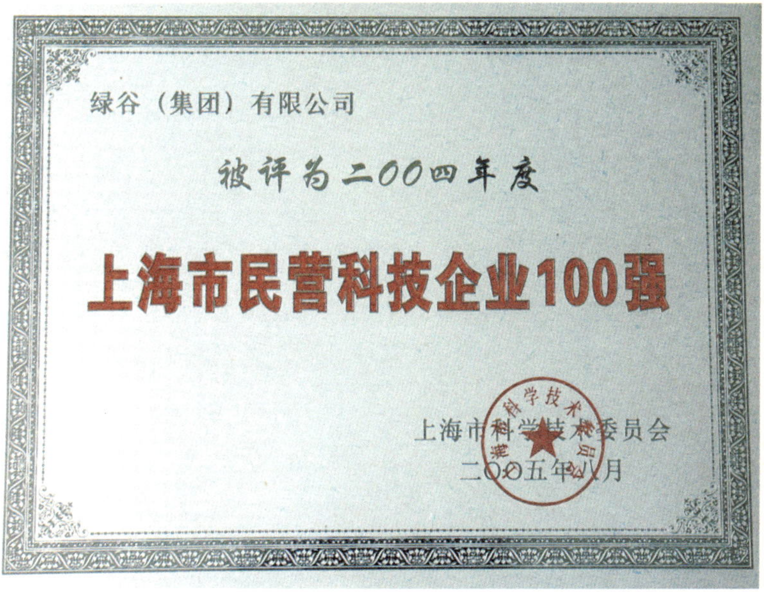

CERTIFICATE AWARDED TO GV AS A TOP 50 INDUSTRIAL ENTERPRISE ACCORDING TO THE SHANGHAI INDUSTRY BUSINESS BUREAU

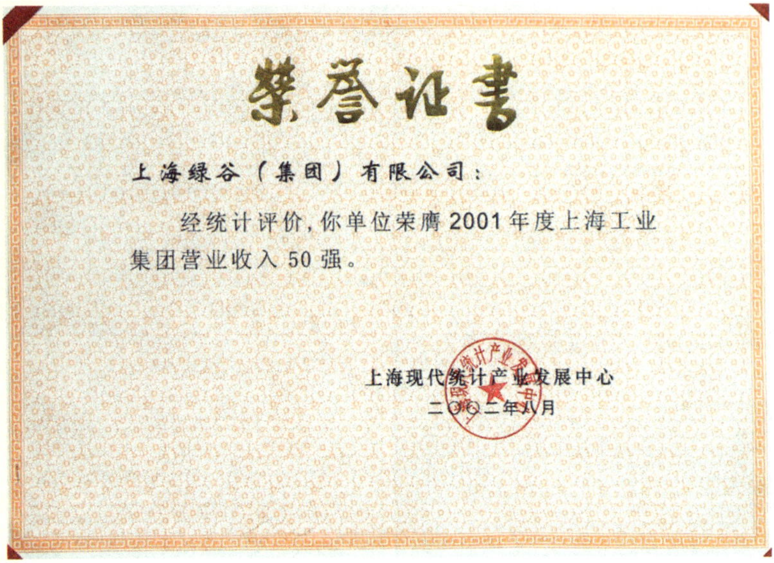

榮譽证書

上海绿谷（集团）有限公司：

经统计评价，你单位荣膺 2001 年度上海工业集团营业收入 50 强。

上海现代统计产业发展中心

二〇〇二年八月

ISO 9002 CERTIFICATE

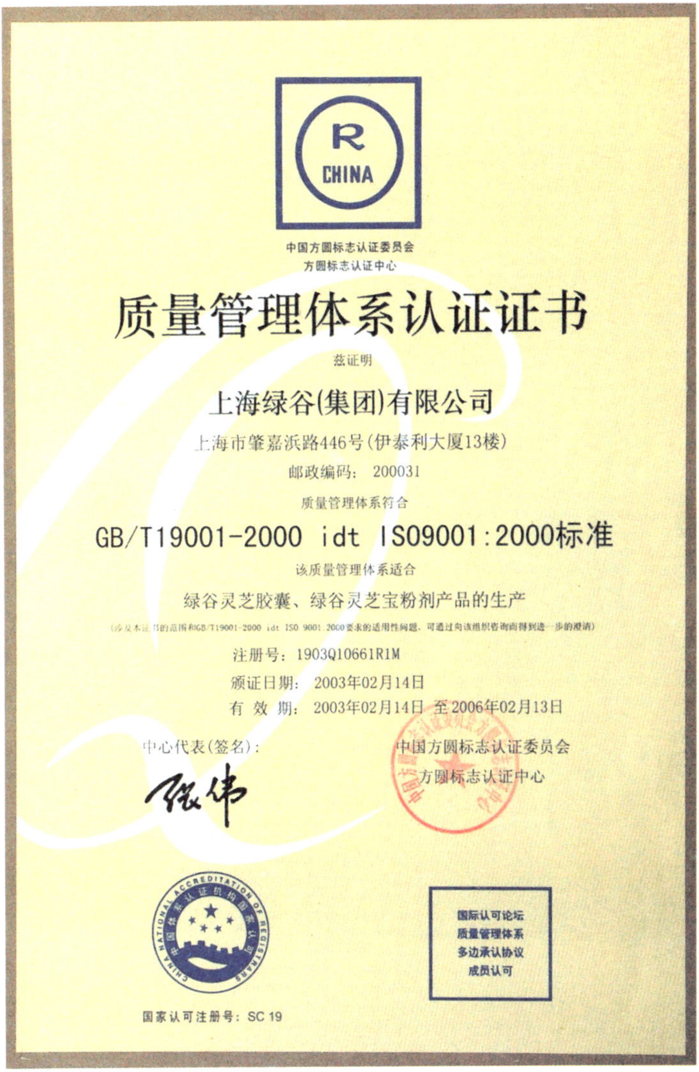

中国方圆标志认证委员会
方圆标志认证中心

质量管理体系认证证书

兹证明

上海绿谷(集团)有限公司

上海市肇嘉浜路446号(伊泰利大厦13楼)

邮政编码：200031

质量管理体系符合

GB/T19001-2000 idt ISO9001:2000标准

该质量管理体系适合

绿谷灵芝胶囊、绿谷灵芝宝粉剂产品的生产

(涉及本证书的范围和GB/T19001-2000 idt ISO 9001:2000要求的适用性问题，可通过向该组织咨询而得到进一步的澄清)

注册号：1903Q10661R1M

颁证日期：2003年02月14日

有 效 期：2003年02月14日 至 2006年02月13日

中心代表(签名)：

中国方圆标志认证委员会
方圆标志认证中心

国际认可论坛
质量管理体系
多边承认协议
成员认可

国家认可注册号：SC 19

GMP CERTIFICATE

中华人民共和国

药品GMP证书

CERTIFICATE OF GOOD MANUFACTURING PRACTICES FOR HUMAN DRUGS
PEOPLE'S REPUBLIC OF CHINA

证书编号: D2010
Certificate No:

企业名称: 西安绿谷制药有限公司
Manufacturer: Xi'an Green Valley Pharmaceutical Co., Ltd.

地　址: 西安市高新技术产业开发区科技一路
Address: Keji 1 Road, Hi-Tech Industrial Development Zone, Xi'an

认证范围: 片剂、胶囊剂、颗粒剂、散剂
Scope of Inspection: Tablets, Capsules, Granules, Powders

经审查，符合中华人民共和国《药品生产质量管理规范》要求。

特发此证。

This is to certify that the above manufacturer Complies with the requirements of Chinese Good Manufacturing Practices.

有效期至 2007 年 12 月 25 日
This certificate remains valid until 25/12/2007

国家药品监督管理局
STATE DRUG ADMINISTRATION
2002 年 12 月 26 日

Issued Date: 26/12/2002

QUALITY ASSURANCE CERTIFICATE

No. L0004

(2001)量认(沪)字(S0124)号

第1页 共2页

上海市药品检验所
药品检验报告书

检验报告专用章

报告书编号：200302146

检品名称	双灵固本散		
批 号	031101	规 格	2g
生产单位或产地	西安绿谷制药有限公司	包 装	复合袋及纸盒
供样单位	西安绿谷制药有限公司	有效期	2005.10
检验目的	委托检验	检品数量	6盒x10袋/盒
检验项目	全项检验	收检日期	11-28-2003
检验依据	国药监局标准试行WS-5407(B-0407)-2002	报告日期	12-04-2003

检验项目	标准规定	检验结果
【性状】	本品应为棕黄色至棕褐色的粉末；气微，味微苦.	本品为棕褐色的粉末；气微，味微苦.
【鉴别】		
(1)显微鉴别	应具“双灵固本散” 的显微特征	具“双灵固本散”的显微特征
(2)化学反应	荧光试验应呈正反应	呈正反应
(3)化学反应	α-萘酚-硫酸试验应呈正反应	呈正反应
(4)化学反应	茚三酮试验应呈正反应	呈正反应
(5)薄层色谱	应具灵芝对照药材的特征斑点	具灵芝对照药材的特征斑点
【检查】		
均匀度	应符合规定	符合规定
水分	不得过9.0%	3.2%

接 下 页

PRODUCT SAFETY TESTING RESULTS

No. L0004

(2001)量认(沪)字(SO124)号

第2页 共2页

上海市药品检验所

药品检验报告书

报告书编号：200302146

检品名称			
批　　号		规　　格	
生产单位或产地		包　　装	
供样单位		有 效 期	
检验目的		检品数量	
检验项目		收检日期	
检验依据		报告日期	

检验项目	标准规定	检验结果
	接 上 页	
装量差异	±7%	符合规定
微生物限度	应符合规定	符合规定
【含量测定】	每袋含灵芝多糖以无水葡萄糖 $[C_6H_{12}O_6]$ 计，不得少于0.14g	0.43g
	以 下 空 白	

结论：　本品按国家药品监督管理局标准（试行）WS-5407(B-0407)-2002检验，结果符合规定.

授权签字人：李[illegible]

APPENDIX 3
Acidic and Alkaline Foods

For optimum health, the human body requires balance, specifically pH balance, between acidic and alkaline foods. Too many acidic foods can cause weight gain, low energy, aches and pains, poor digestion, and even serious illness. According to Chinese physicians, a healthy diet should consist of 30 percent acidic and 70 percent alkaline foods. The following chart provides examples of foods from these two categories.

Acid-forming Foods (30% of diet)

FRUIT

Cranberries

VEGETABLES

Potatoes

GRAINS

Amaranth	Barley
Buckwheat	Corn
Flour	Hemp seed
Kamut	Oats (rolled)
Quinoa	Rice (all)
Rice cakes	Rye
Spelt	Wheat cakes
	Wheat

PROTEIN

Beef	Clams
Fish	Lamb
Lobster	Mussels
Oysters	Pork
Rabbit	Salmon
Shrimp	Scallops
Tuna	Turkey
	Veal

NUTS

Brazil nuts
Pecans
Tahini
Cashews
Peanuts
Walnuts

BEANS & LEGUMES

Almond milk
Chick peas
Kidney beans
Lima beans
Red beans
Soy beans
White beans
Black beans
Green peas
Lentils
Pinto beans
Rice milk
Soy milk

DAIRY PRODUCTS

Butter
Cheese
Milk

FATS & OILS

Avocado oil
Corn oil
Lard
Safflower oil
Canola oil
Flax oil
Olive oil
Sesame oil

DRUGS & CHEMICALS

Aspartame
Hard liquor
Pesticides
Beer
Herbicides
Prescription drugs
Wine

Alkaline-forming Foods (70% of diet)

FRUIT

Apples
Avocados
Berries
Currants
Grapefruits
Apricots
Bananas
Cherries
Dates/Figs
Grapes

Limes	Melons
Nectarines	Oranges
Lemons	Peaches
Pears	Tangerines
Tomatoes	Tropical fruit
	Watermelons

VEGETABLES

Alfalfa	Asparagus
Beets	Broccoli
Brussels sprouts	Cabbages
Carrots	Cauliflowers
Celery	Cucumbers
Eggplants	Garlic
Greens	Lettuces
Mushrooms	Onions
Parsnips	Peas
Peppers	Rutabagas
Sea vegetables	Sprouts
	Squashes

PROTEIN

Chicken breast	Cottage cheese
Eggs (poached)	Millet
Nuts	Seeds
Tempeh	Tofu
Whey protein	Yogurt

SEASONINGS

Chili peppers	Cinnamon
Curry	Ginger
Herbs (al)	Miso
Mustard	Sea salt
Stevia	Tamari

OTHER

Bee pollen	Cider vinegar
Fresh fruit juices	Green juices

Herbal tea
Mineral water
Probiotic cultures
Lecithin
Organic milk
Vegetable juices

Your Notes

Bibliography

Chapter 1

[1] "Cancer Facts & Figures 2005,"American Cancer Society. 19 Jan. 2005. 30 Jan. 2005 <www.cancer.org>.

[2] "Phase 2 Clinical Trial Report of SunRecome for Adjuvant Tumor Treatment." Green Valley Holding Company, Ltd. Shanghai, China, trans. 2004.

[3] Jinshen Chen. "Ganoderma Preparation and Method of Administering." People's Republic of China Patent ZL97106520-9. 16 Sept. 2000.

[4] People's Republic of China SFDA Certificate No. B20020428. March 2002.

[5] *Journal of Clinical Oncology* 2000;18:2505-2521.

[6] "Natural Products Expo West Breaks Prior Records as Community Comes Together." Press release. 24 March 2005. New Hope Natural Media. 10 May 2005. <www.newhope.com>.

[7] "2003 Annual Survey of Hospitals," [latest report]. American Hospital Association. 2003. 8 Feb. 2005. <www.hospitalconnect.com>.

[8] Fareed Zakaria, "Does the Future Belong to China?" *Newsweek,* 9 May 2005. 10 May 2005 <www.newsweek.com>.

Chapter 2

[9] "The Marvelous Mushroom," 11 April 2005 <www.starchefs.com/Features/mushrooms.html>.

[10] "Fungal Biotechnology," 11 April 2005 <www.fungus.org.uk/nwfg/fungbiot.html>.

[11] "A World of Mushrooms," 11 April 2005 <www.knet.co.za/Mushrooms>.

[12] "2004 State of Mushroom Nutrition Research," May 2005. 6 May 2005 <www.mushroomcouncil.org>.

[13] "Medicinal Mushrooms: Their Therapeutic Properties and Current Medical Usage, With Special Emphasis on Cancer Treatments." University Of Strathclyde/Cancer Research UK, May 2002. 6 May 2005 <www.fruiting-bodies.co.uk/cancer_ Research/cr_chapter10.html>.

[14] "Supplements A – Z," 6 May 2005 <www.supplementwatch. com>.

[15] "Medicinal Mushrooms," 2004. 6 May 2005 <www.aloha medicinals.com/mushframes.html>.

[16] Toth, 1983.

Chapter 3

[17] "Reishi Mushroom: Standards of Analysis, Quality Control, and Therapeutics," American Herbal Pharmacopoeia (Santa Cruz, CA) September 2000: 1.

[18] "The Legend of the White Snake," 2005. 28 April 2005 <www.chinapage.com/wsnake.html>.

Chapter 4

[19] Shu-Qian Lin, Sai-Zhen Wang, Zhi-Bin Lin, and Yue-Xin Lin, "Purification and Identification of Glycopeptides from Ganoderma lucidum Fruit Bodies Cultivated with Grass and Wood Logs," *China Traditional Herbal Drugs,* October 2003: 10-872.

Chapter 5

[20] Sasaki T., "Reishi Polysaccharides Contain Anti-tumor Properties," *Chem. Pharm. Bull* 19 (1971): 821.

[21] *Journal of European Pharmacology*, 1989 (or 1990).

[22] *China Oncology Magazine*, 1998.

[23] *Traditional Chinese Medicine*, 1994.

[24] Jinshen Chen, "New Discovery, Pharmacological Function of Ganoderma Extract for Cancer Prevention and Treatment," 1984 (Hong Kong) trans. 2000.

Chapter 6

[25] *Integrated Medical Treatment for Cancer* (Shanghai Green Valley Holding Co., Ltd., of Shanghai, China, 2004).

Chapter 7

[26] Irene S. Levine, Ph.D., "A Dose of Reality, "*Reader's Digest* April 2005: 102-109.

[27] United States, Food and Drug Administration, *Good Manufacturing Practices (GMP)/ Quality System (QS) Regulation.* 1 April 2004. 5 May 2005 <www.fda.gov/cdrh/devadvice/32.html>.

[28] "ISO In Brief: International Standards for a Sustainable World," May 2005. 8 May 2005 <www.iso.org/iso/en/aboutiso/isoinbrief/isoinbrief.html>.

[29] "Just for Kids," 8 May 2005 <www.fungi.com/kids/index.html>.

Chapter 8

[30] "Huang-Qi," NetMateWorld Alternative Medicine, 2001. 16 May 2005 <www.netmatealtmedicine.com/herbs/huang-qi.html>.

[31] "The Treatment of Gastro-Intestinal Cancers with Chinese Medicine," 1 June 2005. 2 June 2005 <www.itmonline.org/Arts/gicancer.html>.

[32] "Helping a Child Cope with Chemo?" 30 June 2003. 18 May 2005 <www.drweil.com>.

[33] "Diagnosis by Pulse," *The Chinese Medicine Sampler,* 2004. 2 June 2005 <www.chinesemedicinesampler.com/diagpulse.html>.

Chapter 9

[34] Reported by Shanghai Green Valley Holding Co., Ltd., of Shanghai, China, 2005.

[35] United States, Department of Health and Human Services, *Median Income for 4-Person Families, by State.* 17 Feb. 2005. 2 June 2005 <www.census.gov/hhes/income4person.html>.

Chapter 10

[36] "About The Lung Cancer Online Foundation," 16 Apr. 2004. 4 June 2005 <www.lungcanceronline.org/foundation/mission.html>.

[37] "Leading Sites of New Cancer Cases and Deaths—2005 Estimates," American Cancer Society, Inc., Surveillance

Research. 2005. 4 June 2005 <www.cancer.org/docroot/MED/content/MED_1_1_Most-Requested_Graphs_And_Figures_2005.asp>.

[38] "Every 12 Minutes," National Breast Cancer Foundation. 2005. 4 June 2005 <www.nationalbreastcancer.org>.

[39] United States, U.S. National Institutes of Health, *Pancreatic Cancer (PDQ®): Treatment.* 20 May 2005. 4 June 2005 <www.cancer.gov/cancerinfo/pdq/treatment/pancreatic/healthprofessional>.

[40] "EIF's NCCRA Emphasizes Educational Efforts for March — National Colorectal Cancer Awareness Month." Press release. 14 March 2005. 5 June 2005 <www.eifoundation.org/national/nccra/press/article2005-03-14.html>.

Chapter 11

[41] "Leading Sites of New Cancer Cases and Deaths—2005 Estimates," American Cancer Society, Inc., Surveillance Research. 2005. 4 June 2005 <www.cancer.org/docroot/MED/content/MED_1_1_Most-Requested_Graphs_And_Figures_2005.asp>.

Glossary

A

Acidic and alkaline foods The human body requires a blood pH of 7.365, which is ideally achieved through a diet containing 30 percent acidic foods (pH >7) and 70 percent alkaline foods (pH<7). Too many acidic foods disrupt this delicate pH balance, which can result in low energy, excess weight, aches and pains, poor digestion, and serious illness. Please see Appendix 3 for a list of acidic and alkaline foods.

Adjuvant therapy Supplementary treatment to reduce the risk that cancer will return. In this book it is revealed that SunRecome is an adjuvant therapy because it improves the effectiveness of radiochemotherapy drugs.

Allopathic medicine The system of medicine, most common in the United States, which is based on the theory that "opposites cure opposites." Allopathic doctors treat diseases with remedies that produce effects differing from those produced by the disease itself. For example, if a patient is constipated, such a doctor might prescribe a medicine that causes diarrhea. Compare to Naturopathic medicine.

Apoptosis The natural cell death process signaled by the nucleus of normally functioning human and animal cells. Cancerous cells are unable to experience the natural cell death process.

B

Beta glucans (or beta-D-glucans) A group of polysaccharides (complex sugars) found in the cell walls of reishi mushrooms and some other plants, best known for their ability to activate immune cells.

Biomarker A pharmacological or physiological measurement used to predict toxicity. For example, prostate health is measured by PSA levels.

C

Chitin (pronounced kīt'in) The hardest natural substance on earth, found in the shells of insects, on crustaceans, and in the flesh of fungi. The hard exterior of reishi spores is made of chitin.

Control Group In a clinical trial, the group that does not receive the experimental drug or substance and is used to compare what happens to the test group(s).

Control medicine A standard, proven treatment for an illness. See Investigational medicine.

Corpulent tongue A term used in Chinese medicine, particularly in regard to tongue diagnosis, to describe a thick, fat, large tongue. These are symptoms of ill health.

Curative Describes the ability of medicine to completely heal the patient. Compare Effective.

Cytology The study of cells.

Cytoprotective drugs Medicines designed to protect cells, such as SunRecome.

D

Decoct To extract the essence of an herb by boiling it for 15 to 20 minutes.

DNA An acronym that stands for deoxyribonucleic acid, the molecule that carries the genetic coding for living organisms. DNA is found inside the nucleus of all cells.

Double-blind testing (also known as a placebo-controlled study) A research procedure in which neither researchers nor patients know who is receiving the experimental substance or treatment and who is receiving the placebo.

E

Eastern medicine The system of healthcare practiced historically in China, which includes herbs, nutritional therapy, restorative physical exercises, meditation, acupuncture and remedial massage.

Effective Describes the ability of a medicine to make the patient feel better or to minimize the side effects of a medication. Compare Curative.

Encapsulated Medicine that is placed in a capsule, as opposed to a loose powder or pill form.

Exacerbation Rapid deterioration of a patient's health.

Extract A solution obtained by steeping or soaking a substance, usually in water or alcohol, to concentrate a desired portion and to eliminate or reduce an undesired portion of the whole substance.

F

FDA Food and Drug Administration; in the United States, a federal agency under the U.S. Department of Health and Human Services established to regulate the release of health-related products and new foods. Many countries have an FDA, including China and Germany.

Fruiting body The above-ground growth of a mushroom, equivalent to the flower of a plant. The fruiting body of a mushroom consists of its stem and cap.

Fu Zheng Therapy A Traditional Chinese Medicinal therapy that combines two or more herbs to help rebuild the body's resistance and its strength so that it can fight off disease. *Ganoderma lucidum* (reishi mushroom) is a traditional Fu Zheng herb, but when highly concentrated it has been proven in clinical studies to outperform combinations of herbs used for cancer therapy.

Fungus (plural: fungi) Latin for "mushroom"; an organism which produce spores (similar to seeds) that can grow into new fungi. Once classified as plants, fungi are now in their own category called the Kingdom Fungi.

G

Ganoderma lucidum The scientific name for reishi mushroom, the most revered herb in Chinese medicine. Common names include ling zhi, lingzhi, ling chih and red reishi.

Germination For a fungus, the process whereby spores sprout and begin to grow.

GMP Short for Good Manufacturing Practice, a system for ensuring that products are consistently produced and controlled according to quality standards. Detailed guidelines have been established by the World Health Organization (WHO). (www.who.int/en/)

Goji (gō-chē′) A tiny red berry, also known as wolfberry or *Lycium barbarum*, that contains the world's richest source of carotenoids, which aid vision and help protect against cataracts, macular degeneration and dry eyes. Goji also contains amino acids, trace minerals, protein, Vitamin C, antioxidants, anti-fungal and anti-bacterial compounds, essential fatty acids, and anti-inflammatory agents.

H

Hematopoiesis The formation of blood or blood cells, especially in bone marrow.

Hermetically sealed Sealed completely airtight.

HPLC A laboratory technique known as High Performance Liquid Chromatography, used to separate substances at high resolutions.

Hypertension High blood pressure.

Hypoallergenic Substances such as medicine, cosmetics, and toiletries which are very unlikely to cause an allergic reaction.

Hypodynamia Diminished strength.

I

Immunology A subfield of biology that deals with the study of antigens and the immune process, and how humans and higher animals fight off disease.

In vitro Latin for "in glass"; biologic techniques or processes performed outside an organism in an artificial environment, such as in a test tube.

In vivo Latin for "in life"; biologic techniques or processes performed within a living organism, such as human clinical testing.

Integrative medicine A system of medicine that combines Eastern and Western medical therapies, not as equal halves, but as is appropriate for each patient.

Investigational medicine An experimental medicine. In clinical trials, one group of patients will be given an experimental drug (the investigational medicine; SunRecome, for example), while the other group will receive either a standard treatment for the illness (the control medicine; ZhenQi Fu Zheng Infusion, for example) or a placebo.

ISO International Organization for Standardization, a worldwide network of more than 150 standards institutes, comprised of one member per country. ISO grants certification to companies that manufacture goods.

L

Lassitude Weariness; fatigue; lack of energy.

M

Metastasis The spread of cancer from its original site to another part of the body via the blood or lymphatic systems.

Moxibustion A TCM technique which predates acupuncture. In moxibustion therapy, the mugwort herb is aged, ground, fluffed and burned or otherwise processed into a stick resembling a cigar and used directly on the skin to stimulate circulation thus promoting healing.

Mycelium The initial growth of a fungus via fermentation (in a tank full of liquid) or on a natural substrate.

Mycoinfoostasis Whole-body balance, with a natural resistance to disease.

Mycologist A person who studies fungi professionally. The term derives from the Greek word *mykes*, which means "mushroom."

N

Naturopathic medicine An integration of herbal medicine, acupuncture, bodywork, dietary therapy and exercise based on Traditional Chinese Medicine principles.

O

Oncology The branch of medicine concerned with the study and treatment of tumors.

P

Palliative effect A treatment that improves a patient's quality of life but does not cure the disease.

Pallid countenance Pale, unhealthy skin color; lacking in vitality.

Parametric and non-parametric tests Standard statistical tests used to verify the results of a study, including Chi-square, Ridit and Adopt *t*-test.

Pathology The branch of medical science that studies the causes, nature and effects of diseases.

pH A measure of acid and alkaline balance. The abbreviation pH stands for "potential of Hydrogen." See Acidic and Alkaline Foods.

Pharmacology The science or study of drug preparation, properties, uses and effects.

Photographology The study of photography.

Placebo A substance which is designed to have no pharmacological effect on the test subject of a clinical trial. See Investigational medicine.

Polysaccharide Any of many carbohydrates that are made up of chains of simple sugars. The reishi mushroom contains more than 50 polysaccharides, which can stimulate the entire immune system to fight off invading cancer cells.

Proprietary Protected by patent, trademark or copyright.

PSA index A blood test that measures an enzyme called "prostate specific antigen" (PSA) to help diagnose prostate cancer.

Q

Qi Vital energy; vitality, as defined by Traditional Chinese Medicine.

Qigong A Chinese exercise routine consisting of controlled breathing, focused concentration and simple movements.

R

Radiochemotherapy Cancer treatments consisting of both radiation therapy and chemotherapy.

S

SFDA China's Food and Drug Administration. The "S" stands for "Sino," which means "China."

Spawn A transplanted fungus.

Spectrophotometer A machine used to measure how much light of a given wavelength is absorbed by a liquid sample, or to measure how intense (bright) the spectral lines and bands produced by the sample are, relative to each other.

Spiritlessness Lacking general enthusiasm.

Spores The microscopic, seed-like component of a fungus, released from under its cap, that contains its reproductive potential.

Substrate The surface on which an organism, such as the reishi mushroom, grows or is attached, including wood logs, wood pulp, rice, corn, soybean stalks, wheat straw, corncobs, cottonseed or lotus-seed shells or wild grass.

T

Tai chi A Chinese martial art, characterized by soft, slow, precise yet flowing movements used for stress release and immune system health.

Telomerase An enzyme present in rapidly dividing cells, such as in tumors. Telomeres shorten whenever a cell divides; when the telomeres become very small, the cell stops dividing.

Test Group In a clinical study, the group that receives the experimental substance, such as SunRecome.

Triterpene A medicinally valuable compound of the reishi mushroom. Certain triterpenes have been proven to slow the growth of cancer enzymes.

Thready pulse A thin, weak pulse.

Topoisomerase enzymes Enzymes that are critical to the normal functioning of any living cell.

Tremella A nutritious jelly fungus and a staple in Chinese health food cooking and in Asian beauty supplements; used to nourish the stomach, moisten the lungs, and make skin soft, moist and pliable.

W

WBC count A blood test to measure the number of white blood cells. A WBC count >500 places a patient at risk for a fatal infection; a WBC count <30,000 indicates a massive infection or a serious disease.

Western medicine Medicine practiced by medical doctors (M.D.) or doctors of osteopathy (D.O.); also called "allopathy." See Allopathic medicine.

WHO The acronym for the World Health Organization of the United Nations, which coordinates international health activities and helps governments improve health services.

Y

Yin and Yang In Traditional Chinese Medicine, the two groups into which human organs are categorized. Yin organs are substantial, passive and solid: the heart, spleen, lungs, kidney and liver. Yang organs are functional and hollow, where foods and fluids pass through: the small intestine, stomach, large intestine and bladder. According to TCM theory, imbalance between Yin and Yang is the cause of disease.

Resources

Mycology Information, Societies and Clubs

American Mushroom Institute (AMI), (202) 842-4344; www.americanmushroom.org

Mycological Society of America, www.msafungi.org

North American Mycological Association (NAMA), (503) 657-7358; www.namyco.org

WWW Virtual Library of Mycology, http://mycology.cornell.edu

National Alternative Health

National Center for Complementary and Alternative Medicine, (888) 644-6226; www.nccam.nih.gov

National Cancer Support

American Cancer Society, (800) ACS-2345; www.cancer.org

SunRecome and Reishi Capsule Distributors

7 Day Health Corporation, (626) 968-9420; *info@7dayhealth.com*. For online orders, please go to www.alternative2cancer.com for SunRecome and to www.goldvitamins.com for reishi capsule orders.

China Only – Green Valley Holding Co., Ltd., 0086-21-50809727; *sun@sunrecome.com*; www.green-valley.com

Notes

Index

ORDER FORM

China's Cancer Solution

$16.95
($14.95 includes tax, plus $2.00 ground shipping)

Please send __ copy(s) of *China's Cancer Solution* to...

NAME ____

ADDRESS ____

CITY ____

STATE __________________________ZIP CODE ________________

ENCLOSED IS MY CHECK FOR $ _______________

❑ $16.95 per book, which includes tax and ground shipping (7-10 days) anywhere in the U.S.

❑ $19.95 per book for delivery within the U.S. in 2 to 3 days

For international delivery or questions, please send an e-mail to reishi@7dayhealth.com

Please make check payable to:
7 Day Health

Send to: 7 Day Health Publishing
2862 Antisana Place
Hacienda Heights, CA USA 91745

Book orders may also be placed online at:
www.alternative2cancer.com